Living Day To Day With Severe Osteoporosis

What Every Person Should Know Regardless of Age

Alice V. Roberts

Bloomington, IN 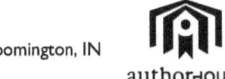 Milton Keynes, UK

authorHOUSE®

AuthorHouse™
1663 Liberty Drive, Suite 200
Bloomington, IN 47403
www.authorhouse.com
Phone: 1-800-839-8640

AuthorHouse™ UK Ltd.
500 Avebury Boulevard
Central Milton Keynes, MK9 2BE
www.authorhouse.co.uk
Phone: 08001974150

First published by AuthorHouse 9/14/2007

ISBN: 978-1-4259-7067-3 (sc)

Library of Congress Control Number: 2007902748

Printed in the United States of America
Bloomington, Indiana

This book is printed on acid-free paper.

THIS BOOK IS DEDICATED TO

This book is dedicated to my husband Randy, who married me despite my disabilities and is a better caregiver than I am a patient. His continued support cannot be appreciated enough. To my daughters Karen and Laura, who were so helpful during my recoveries. And finally, this is also dedicated to my parents for all their love and concerns.

Wishes and dreams are merely idle thoughts.
You cannot succeed unless you try.
Alice V. Roberts

ACKNOWLEDGEMENTS

To everyone who supported me when I said I was writing this book, I thank you. I had a dream; I wanted to be heard and make difference concerning osteoporosis and you supported me in that. I will be forever grateful.

I must include friends that are truly treasured: Michelle Ashley, Bobby D'Avignon and Bette Jo (B.J.) Lytle. They have always been there to help at any time.

Thank you to my doctors at the Sedona Medical Center in Sedona, Arizona, and the Mayo Clinic in Scottsdale, Arizona. And to Phil Sowers, the physical therapist that discovered I had osteoporosis on the afternoon when I went in for migraine relief.

Thank you to my editor, Sandi Greene, for all of her help. And finally to Sergeant Brian Andrews, Sergeant Ralph O'Donnal, and Animal Control Officer Teri Moore, a few of my former co-workers at the Camp Verde Marshal's Office where I worked until leaving on medical disability. They could not have been more helpful as I continued working with injuries that limited my capabilities. I appreciated all of their help and support.

The entire time I was researching and writing this book, my Siamese cat Pywacket was on my desk. She was my constant shadow and supervisor. And occasionally when she would hit the keyboard with her paw I would click "undo" and keep on typing.

Living Day To Day With Severe Osteoporosis

What Every Person Should Know Regardless of Age

I have written this true story about myself for every person regardless of age. If only one person can prevent severe osteoporosis from happening to them then this book was worth writing.

I am not a doctor, nor do I have any experience in the medical field. I am not attempting to imply a medical diagnosis or recommend treatment for anyone reading this book. Instead, this is a story of my medical plight with severe osteoporosis. It explains what osteoporosis is, how I acquired the disease, and what it is has done to my life. It is also to encourage every man and woman to examine his or her life, and do something about this bone disease before it is too late.

I encourage you to examine your age, diet, health, and lifestyle. If you are a woman, ask your doctor for a bone density test whether you are still having monthly periods or have had either a partial or complete hysterectomy. Do it regardless of any estrogen replacement you may be taking. It can mean the difference in how you conduct your daily routine for the rest of your life. When I was diagnosed, once the damage was done — it was done! I know. I am living with the damage and restrictions now. I was diagnosed at age 35. When I turned 49 my world literally crashed out from under me.

Fortunately today, there are options out there to help build bone back up. So please read this book carefully. See your doctor and ask for a bone density test immediately. Start helping yourself before it is too late. It is important for you and your family.

Chapter 1

To better understand the journey this book takes, it is important to know what osteoporosis is. As I share details about my personal health — and why my life is at the stage it is now with this disease — it is frightening to think how many people may read this and find it to be a story about them too.

How I, along with millions of others, became a victim of osteoporosis will be revealed in detail later in this book. Throughout this book I will discuss extensively what osteoporosis is, how I was diagnosed, how I was treated, and the changes it has made in my day-to-day living as a result of this disease.

The National Institute of Health - Osteoporosis and Related Bone Diseases say osteoporosis has been defined as a disease where there is a loss of bone mass and structural deterioration of the bone tissue. It is described as a loss of calcium to the bone and makes the individual more susceptible to breaking bones. The hips, ribs, spine, and wrists are the higher risk areas for breakage, but any bone can be affected. Compression fractures of the spine can lead to deterioration of support from the vertebrae resulting in a stooped back (hunched over) and/or height loss. As bones become weaker with age, the risk of osteoporosis becomes even greater. Once a debilitating disease known mostly for afflicting the elderly, men and women regardless of their age can and do become victims.

Over ten million people currently have osteoporosis. Over triple that amount of people have a low bone mass. People with a low bone mass are more susceptible to osteoporosis. Osteoporosis is responsible for over one and a half million fractures a year. This includes 300,000 hip fractures, 250,000 wrist fractures, 700,000 vertebrae fractures, and more than 300,000 fractures at other sites. Estimated national direct expenditures, (hospitals and nursing homes) for osteoporosis and related fractures is over twenty billion dollars a year.

The first 20 years of life are critical to bone formation. At that point it then becomes important to prevent bone loss. Anything that prevents healthy bone formation or bone structure can lead to fragile bones and osteoporosis. Exercise is important. Not only does it improve bone health, it also increases muscle strength, coordination and balance, and leads to better overall health.

Bone formation during the growing years and the level of exercise are among the important factors in creating healthy bones. Bone is living, growing tissue. It is made mostly of collagen (a protein that provides a soft framework) and calcium phosphate (a mineral that adds strength and hardens the framework). This combination of collagen and calcium makes bones strong, yet flexible to withstand stress. More than 99% of the body's calcium is contained in the bones and teeth. The remaining 1% is found in the blood.

Menopause is the number one cause of osteoporosis. Certain risk factors have also been linked to people with osteoporosis. There are, however, people who have osteoporosis and show no signs of those risk factors. Some risk factors can be changed and some cannot. Risk factors a person can change include hormone levels (low estrogen for women and low testosterone in men), calcium and vitamin D intake, caffeine intake, excessive alcohol use (affects the body's ability to absorb calcium), smoking (decreases calcium absorption in the intestines), exercise, rest, and certain medications. Risk factors that cannot be changed are age (menopause increases bone loss), surgical menopause (especially if the ovaries are removed), body size (small boned women are more susceptible), national origin (those of Asian and Caucasian decent have a higher risk of getting osteoporosis), family history (parents with a medical history of osteoporosis or fractures), and sex (as previously mentioned, women have a greater chance of developing osteoporosis).

Depending on the severity of osteoporosis, there can be mild discomfort or constant pain, especially to the lower back region. A person can sustain fractures that can leave them permanently handicapped. They may not be able to function without the assistance of a cane, crutches, walker, wheelchair, or electric scooter. When ribs are broken there is always the scare of puncturing a lung, which can be very serious.

One out of every two women will have an osteoporosis related fracture sometime after the age of 50. Approximately 25% of the women over the age of 50 who fracture a hip will need long-term nursing care. Over half of the women who fracture a hip due to osteoporosis will not be able to walk without assistance. Additionally, approximately 25% who have a hip fracture die within one year (fortunately I have not broken a hip yet). One out of eight men will experience a fracture due to osteoporosis. One-third of hip fractures suffered by men are related to osteoporosis, and one-third of these men die within the first year after the fracture. Obviously, osteoporosis has become a major health threat for millions of men and women.

In my case, some of my fractures have required surgery and extensive physical therapy to regain the use of a limb. My last fracture left me with approximately 80% mobility to my right leg. It will never improve, and that is just from one fracture. During several fractures I was confined to a wheelchair before graduating to a walker, then crutches, followed by a cane. I am now supposed to use a cane or walker all the time and I have a permanent handicap placard for my vehicle.

Doctors have told me my next fracture may be the one that could break my back or neck leaving me partially or permanently paralyzed. Every time I fall I try to watch how I go down. I tell myself to break an arm or leg but protect the back and neck. Yet, when you fall, it happens so quickly you hardly have time to think. I fall often because my muscles are weak and the bones are thin. I will be walking and the next thing I know, my leg has given out and down I go. At any given time if an x-ray was taken of my spine there would be approximately a thousand hairline cracks. I am supposed to swim everyday for the rest of my life. Swimming is supposed to strengthen the muscles to help prevent falls and to protect the bones when I do fall. It can mean the difference in paralysis if and when I fall.

In December of 2004, my employer required a medical update because of my physical limitations. A bone mineral density test was done and my osteoporosis was so much worse that I was considered a medical and financial risk for any employer. I was always in pain and knew the results would be bad; I just did not think it would be that bad.

I began short-term disability at the end of December 2004. After six months, beginning in June 2005, I was approved for long-term disability, and told it could take up to six months for payments to begin. The payments would be retroactive, meaning I would receive pay effective June 1st to the present. Fortunately, my first check arrived within two weeks of applying and being approved.

Friends have asked how I live with all of this. My response is that falling and broken bones have become a way of life for me. I cannot change what has happened. I can only try to recover from a fracture and make the most of what I can do.

When I first learned I had to go on disability I had a six-week "pity party" for myself. I had no desire to get out of bed — there was no reason to. I was not able to go to work. I kept asking myself, "Why me?" I had just turned 49 and my first grandchild was about to celebrate his first birthday. Then one day I realized there must be more awareness concerning osteoporosis.

Something positive had to come from this. I needed to become a voice speaking out on this disease. I needed to write a book, speak on talk shows, and develop a local community support group. People need to know the warning signs I discuss in this book. And when I mentioned all this to my doctor at the Mayo Clinic he thought it was a fantastic idea and wished me luck. He also said there is not enough education or awareness on this disease and any exposure would certainly help the cause.

There are so many options available today to help slow down bone loss. There are even medications to help rebuild bones. Unfortunately, 25 years ago the medical field did not have the extensive knowledge that they do today regarding the causes of osteoporosis and its treatment. When that little neon sign is flashing do not ignore it. You can do something about it if you take action soon enough. Do not let your bones become like mine.

The National Institute of Health - Osteoporosis and Related Bone Diseases say each year that osteoporosis causes hundreds of vertebral fractures, also known as compression or crush fractures. Vertebrae, which form the bony spine and hold the back upright, are called cervical in the neck area, thoracic in the middle back area, and lumbar in the waist and lower back. While fractures can occur anywhere in the spine, they are most common in the middle or thoracic area of the back[1].

Picture of Healthy Bone[1]

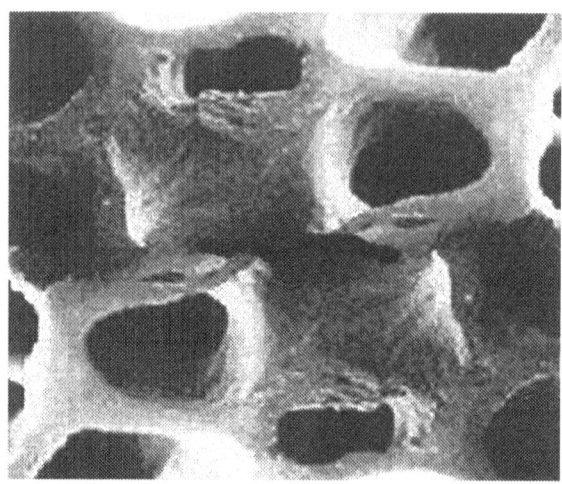

Picture of Bone with Osteoporosis[2]

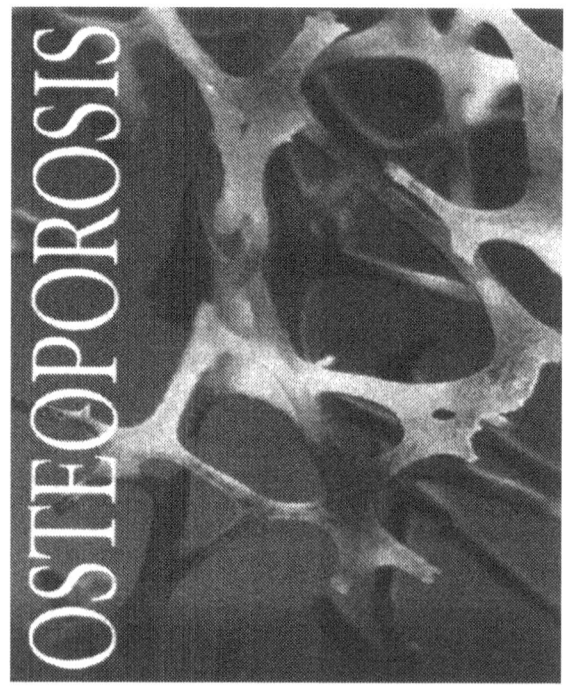

[1,2] Photo courtesy of National Institute of Health-Osteoporosis and Related Bone Disease

The following chart shows how bones change with age. It shows the change in posture with age as compression fractures lead to spinal deterioration of the vertebrae resulting in a stooped back and height loss.

How Bones Change as You Age[3]

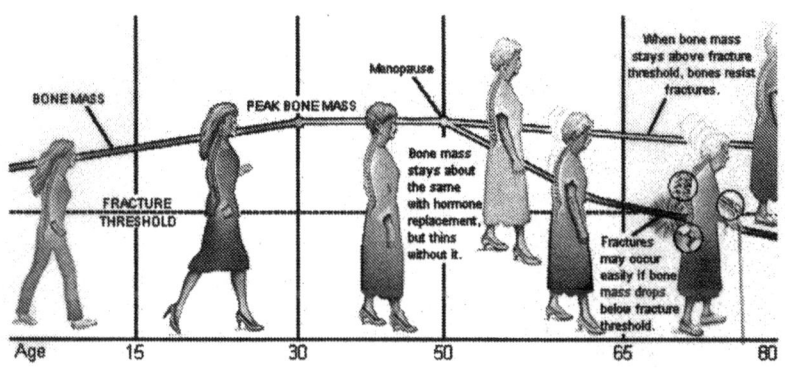

[3] Chart courtesy of Lee J. Monlezun, Jr. M.D. FACOG

Chapter 2

At the age of 24, I had severe endometriosis and had to have a total hysterectomy (removal of the cervix, fallopian tubes, ovaries and uterus). So at this early age I began menopause. In 1991, at the age of 35, doctors at the Mayo Clinic in Scottsdale, Arizona, diagnosed me with significant osteoporosis. A bone mineral density (BMD) test had been performed, and the results showed a bone density of only 67%. I was told that my osteoporosis was related to premature menopause, poor calcium intake, lack of Vitamin D supplements, family history, and because I had been completely intolerant to estrogen supplements.

It is amazing how most of my medical problems were and still are intertwined so much to lead to this result of osteoporosis. As a child I suffered from migraine headaches beginning at the age of three. It was always accompanied with nausea and vomiting. I went through numerous tests to rule out tumors and various diseases. The doctors thought the migraines might possibly go away when I began my monthly menstrual cycles. My parents and I were told that sometimes a change in hormone levels could reduce migraine headaches.

As a pre-teen, I began my menstrual cycles early around eleven and a half years old. They were always extremely painful with a tremendous flow that lasted seven to ten days (so much for the three to five days you learned about in school). As I got older they became even worse. By the time I was in high school I was getting my assignments so that I could spend the first couple of days in bed with my feet elevated up high. This became a monthly routine along with each period. I attended a private school so staying home each month was not a major problem considering the circumstances. The headaches not only didn't disappear, but they actually worsened and coincided with my periods.

My mother and I shared the same symptoms during our monthly periods but hers were much worse and she was older. When I was 13, my mother had a complete hysterectomy because of endometriosis at the age of 45. At that time endometriosis had been described to me as the lining of the uterus called the endometrium, growing outside of the uterus.

As my teenage years continued to pass I experienced more painful periods. Because of constant clots and heavy flows, my physical activities were limited at the doctor's request. I was experiencing hemorrhaging, became anemic, and had to take iron supplements. When I was 16, I saw the gynecologist who had performed the hysterectomy on my mother. He felt that I too, had endometriosis and surgery might be an option to seriously consider despite my young age. Plus, the only true way to confirm that I had endometriosis would have required explorative surgery. I, however, wanted to eventually become a mother, so it was decided I would continue bed rest with each monthly period and restrict physical activity during those times. If things became much worse, then the situation would have to be re-evaluated. Believe it or not, all these problems and more led up to my osteoporosis.

After graduating from high school I headed off to college attending Northern Arizona University in Flagstaff, Arizona. Flagstaff was at an altitude of approximately 6,700 feet above sea level. Little did I know that high altitudes could affect your monthly period. At this point, mine went totally out of control, and they never stopped. If they did stop it was only for about five days then they would continue again for another 20 to 25 days.

I finally saw a gynecologist in Flagstaff who put me on a birth control pill. This was done in hopes of getting my periods back on a regular cycle. It did help, in fact my period would last only five to six days. They were still as painful and heavy in flow, but the duration was shorter. I thought I could handle this and decided to stick with it.

Two years after starting college I was married at the age of 20 and made Flagstaff my permanent hometown. After three months of marriage I became pregnant but miscarried in the first eight weeks. I was told that was quite common with first pregnancies, especially if monthly periods were difficult. I did not know if that was true or not, that's just what my doctor told me. Soon after, I became pregnant again. I had more than the usual morning sickness and was hospitalized for dehydration several times. I had also experienced cramping and bleeding which was not considered normal before giving birth. My mother came out from Los Angeles to help me. On her first visit she noticed I was not acting normal, asked what medication I was given for nausea and immediately called my husband home from work to rush us to the hospital. I was taking Compazine and she had recognized the symptoms because she too was allergic to Compazine. My throat and tongue were swelling up and I was having uncontrollable neck spasms. By the time we arrived at the emergency room my eyes were rolling back. Amazingly, as the doctor intravenously injected a medication for the allergic reaction I could feel myself going back to normal — it was that instantaneous.

I did not know it at that time, but a lack of tolerance and reaction to various medications would help lead to my osteoporosis. It also would stand in the way of treatment.

I was soon going to learn that I had endometriosis. What I did not know was that it would be a key factor in causing my osteoporosis.

After having gone through the pregnancy and giving birth to a healthy baby girl, my periods became even worse. The cramps were almost unbearable with numerous clots and very heavy flow. Intimacy with my husband became extremely painful. I also had a lot of lower back and pelvic pain whether I was having a period or not. The migraines, too, had become even worse, requiring an injection of medication for both pain and vomiting. The doctor usually gave me Demerol for the pain and Vistaril for the nausea. I was then able to sleep off the headache and by the next morning it would be gone.

The Office of Women's Health in the Department of Health and Human Services says that endometriosis is a result of the lining of the uterus known as endometrium growing outside of the uterus. It is mostly found in the pelvic cavity, usually in one or more of these places: on or under the ovaries, behind the uterus, on tissue that holds the uterus in place, or on the bowels or bladder. As the tissue grows, it can develop growths (tumors or implants) that are usually benign (non-cancerous). The growths can cause mild to severe pain. Endometriosis can distort the pelvic area and may even cause infertility (not being able to get pregnant). Women who have suffered from endometriosis may also be more prone to experience reactions or intolerance to certain medications that would demand they discontinue their use.

A common symptom of endometriosis is pain that is mostly located in the abdomen, lower back, and pelvic areas. Chronic pain includes both the lower back and pelvis. During menstrual periods, one may experience heavier than normal flows, extremely painful menstrual cramps that may worsen over time, and painful urination and bowel movements. There can also be mild discomfort to extreme pain during and after sexual intercourse. Premenstrual spotting or bleeding between periods is quite common as well.

Today there are ways of determining if a woman has endometriosis. The most common is a laparoscopy, which is a surgical procedure done under general anesthesia, where a narrow scope with a light is placed inside the abdominal cavity. This allows the surgeon to see any growths or tissues resulting from endometriosis. This procedure shows the location, extent, and size of the growths if endometriosis is present. A doctor can feel fairly certain a patient suffers from endometriosis from the symptoms they are experiencing, but there is no guarantee that is what the patient really has without actually seeing it. Today, for women suffering from endometriosis, doctors can offer more options than just a total hysterectomy, thereby stalling the onset of menopause and eventually osteoporosis, which leads to longer and healthier lives.

In early 1978, when I was 22, I began experiencing violent pain on my right side around the area where my right ovary was located. One night around three in the morning it was so bad I was taken to the emergency room of the local hospital. By now my obstetrician/gynecologist knew my medical history. The next thing I knew I was headed to surgery. When I came to I was told abdominal surgery had been done. My right ovary had a ruptured cyst the size of a grapefruit. The cyst had been removed but the right fallopian tube was damaged. The doctor had attempted to repair the tube, but could not guarantee its success. I had severe endometriosis. The doctor also thought I probably only had one year to get pregnant again, if even that long. Finally, the doctor had told me the growth could cause infertility.

Affecting a vastly large number of women each year, endometriosis can be hereditary and has no age boundaries. Severe endometriosis causes scarring and can damage the fallopian tubes — just as it had done to my right one. Ovarian cysts are quite common. Again, just like the one removed from my right ovary.

Back in 1978, before this knowledge, all of my problems were still leading up to osteoporosis. Approximately six weeks after having the surgery I experienced an awful leg cramp in my left leg in the middle of the night. I rubbed the hell out of it not knowing that was never to be done. Later in the night I could not breathe so I kept hitting my husband in the chest as I gasped for air. I had also experienced sharp chest pains and horrible sweating. My husband called the operator since 911 was not in existence at that time and the police arrived before the fire and ambulance. The policeman put oxygen on me and I began to feel better. Once the medics arrived, the head medic said I had hyperventilated. He had already had two cases of that in the same night and left with me breathing in a brown bag. The medic made his own diagnosis without even calling in to the hospital.

The next morning my chest was still in pain every time I inhaled and exhaled so I called my internist who sent me to the hospital for a lung scan after hearing the events from the previous night and knowing I had surgery just six weeks ago. The lung scan showed a blood clot also known as a pulmonary embolism that I should have died from according to the size and location.

The lung scan was done by injecting a contrast dye in to my vein; making the clot more visible in an x-ray. That allowed the doctor to see the location and size of the blood clot.

Apparently the clot was rather large and it was only by some great miracle I was still alive. I never left the hospital, but was admitted for two weeks on complete bed rest (including a bed pan) and given heavy doses of Coumadin, a blood thinner that reduces clots.

My doctor had explained to me that a pulmonary embolism occurs when a blood clot travels to the lungs and blocks the pulmonary artery, thereby blocking the blood flow from the heart (which can be fatal). Since I was recovering from surgery and somewhat immobile, that cramp in my leg had been a clot in a vein. When I rubbed it like I did (not knowing it was a clot), it shot right up in to my lung.

Once I was released to go home, I remained on the Coumadin for six months having weekly blood tests to check my clotting time. The biggest precaution was to not cut myself for fear that I could bleed to death.

Since that happened, every time I have major surgery I am put on Coumadin for eight weeks as well as checking the clotting time weekly with a routine blood test. Depending on the results, the doctor can increase or decrease the dosage. As for the medic who had made his own diagnosis that evening; he was taken before a review board for not following protocol. His reprimand was that he was unable to practice for three months. He would have lost his job if I had died that night.

My husband and I tried and hoped for another pregnancy but it just was not happening. The headaches were horrible and so were the periods. I felt helpless taking care of my young daughter, and many times a babysitter came in when my husband was at work. All these problems had become quite debilitating.

Finally, I thought I was pregnant but I was also having a horrendous migraine. The doctor insisted I come in for a shot. But when I got there I told him I thought I was pregnant (because of morning sickness) so they did blood work to see if I was. It came out negative, and I was given the shot and my husband drove me home. The next day my OB/GYN called and said time had run out and we needed to do a total hysterectomy. I still swore I was pregnant — a woman just knows. I knew my body. I had been through a lot. The doctor, on the other hand said I had convinced myself I was pregnant and that was the reason for the morning sickness.

The surgery was scheduled but I did not show up. After all, I kept insisting I was pregnant. I did receive a letter from the hospital administrator telling me I had been irresponsible and inconsiderate. And a bill for the operating room and staff that was scheduled for my surgical procedure was included. Before my OB/GYN called me into his office to lecture me on missing the surgery, he did another test and it confirmed I was pregnant. I asked for a copy of the test results, which I mailed to that hospital administrator. I know he received my paperwork because I did not get a letter from him but I did get a bill that showed a zero balance. It terrified me to think I could have lost that baby if I had gone through with the surgery.

Since I was definitely pregnant there was a new set of rules to live by. I had to be very careful in my activities. I could not lift my daughter, or do anything that could strain me in any way at all. I still experienced morning sickness but a different nausea medication helped with that issue.

About ten weeks into the pregnancy I started bleeding and continued to do so until I delivered. Apparently the placenta was partially detached. My OB/GYN had me seen by a local fertility/infertility specialist. At first they thought I might have to abort the baby; that neither of us would survive. The doctors eventually firmly believed I would make it but the baby probably would not survive.

Determined to have this baby, I was put on bed rest for the remainder of the pregnancy. When my husband left for work a wonderful babysitter came. She took care of our daughter, did laundry, cleaning, and groceries. The sitter even took our daughter to her family dinners and barbeques. Our sitter's family became our daughter's second family. My mother came out again but not as much since we had a fulltime sitter. I did a lot of reading and needlepoint during those long months in bed. I was allowed out of bed to eat, shower, use the bathroom and see my doctor. If any changes occurred in the pregnancy those privileges would end. The migraine headaches were continuous throughout the pregnancy. In fact, it was one very, very long migraine. I was also taking different medications for headaches and nausea. Vomiting was not an option. There were numerous hospitalizations throughout the pregnancy to monitor the baby's and my health.

Eventually at the age of 24, in April of 1980, the day came and I went in to labor. It lasted exactly eight hours, which was the same as the first pregnancy. Because of the seriousness involved, both my OB/GYN and the pediatrician left their offices and arrived at the hospital when I did. The two doctors did not want to waste any precious time in driving so they sat there and played cards until the delivery. As soon as my new daughter was born, she was taken to a special unit to be assessed for any serious complications.

Once I was back in my room I wanted to see her but was told it would be a while. I was convinced she had not survived and everyone was afraid to tell me. I told them I had expected the worst but hoped for the best and could handle it. They kept insisting she was alive but until I saw her I would not believe them. So they put me in a wheelchair and took me to her. She truly was a miracle. She had survived. They said they would bring her to my room in a few hours. The pediatrician wanted to be sure of everything first.

Because of all the medications taken during and after the pregnancy, nursing was not an option. My new baby had been born at 8:30 in the evening and at 6:00 the next morning I was in surgery. My doctor performed a tubal ligation as a precaution until a complete hysterectomy could be performed. The doctor wanted to wait about six months and give my body time to heal from the pregnancy and delivery. I was 24 years old, had two daughters and was ready to do it — no more arguments from me.

Female Reproductive System[4]

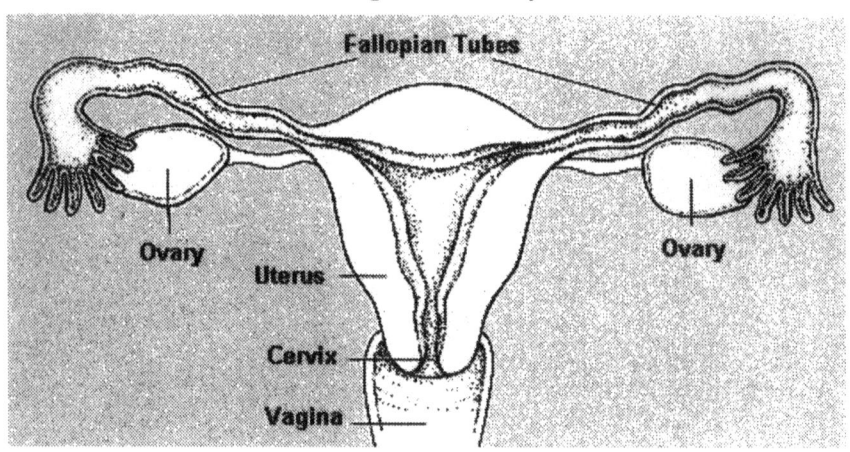

What Endometriosis Looks Like[5]

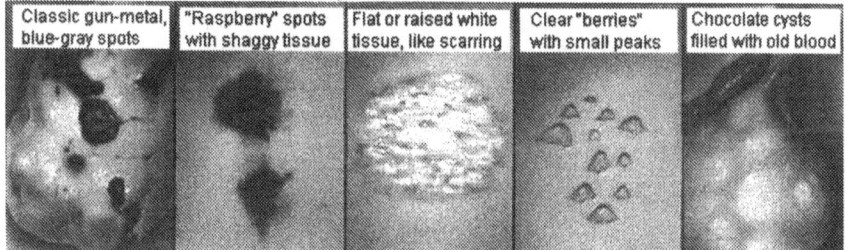

The Stages of Endometriosis[6]

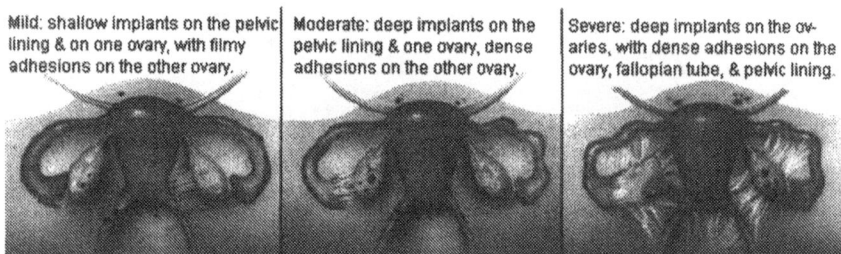

Mine was scarred and was very severe)

[4,5,6] Courtesy of Lee J. Monlezun, Jr., M.D. FACOG

Tubal Ligation Prior to Cut[7]

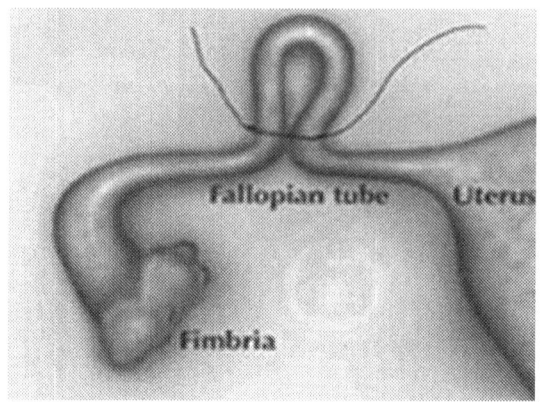

Fallopian Tubes Tied and Cut[8]

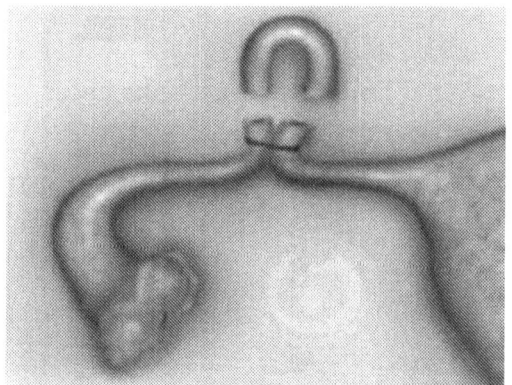

Final Results[9]

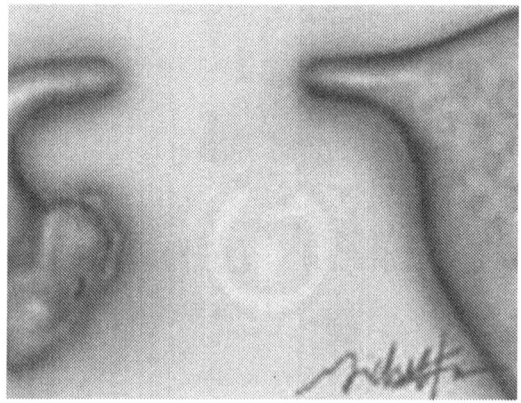

[7,8,9] Courtesy of Chapel Hill Tubal Reversal Center.
http://www.tubal-reversal.net

Chapter 3

According to the Office of Women's Health, a hysterectomy — the second most common surgery among women — is an operation to remove a woman's uterus (the womb where a baby grows during pregnancy). Depending on the medical reason for surgery, sometimes the cervix, fallopian tubes, and ovaries are removed when the uterus is removed. If a woman has not reached menopause at the time of her hysterectomy, she will no longer have a monthly period or be able to get pregnant.

If the ovaries are removed before a woman has had a chance to reach natural menopause, the sudden loss of her main source of female hormones will cause her to suddenly enter menopause (surgical menopause). This can cause more severe symptoms than natural menopause.

The cervix is the lower end of the uterus. The ovaries are organs that produce eggs and hormones. The fallopian tubes carry the eggs from the ovaries to the uterus. The type of hysterectomy that is necessary depends on what is removed.

There are several types of hysterectomies. A complete or total hysterectomy (the most common) removes the cervix as well as the uterus. A partial or subtotal hysterectomy removes the upper part of the uterus and leaves the cervix in place. And a radical hysterectomy removes the uterus, the cervix, and the upper part of the vagina and supporting tissue (this is usually done in the case of cancer). Often one or both fallopian tubes and ovaries are removed at the time of the hysterectomy. Hysterectomies are often done for the following reasons:

- Uterine Fibroids: Non-cancerous tumors that grow in the muscle of the uterus.
- Endometriosis: The lining of the uterus begins to grow outside of the uterus and on nearby organs.
- Uterine Prolapse: A benign condition in which the uterus moves from its usual place down in to the vagina.

There are various alternatives to having a hysterectomy but it depends on a woman's medical history and if any alternative option was available or successful. Patients are often treated with hormones to lower their estrogen level. A hysterectomy becomes the last resort.

It was a rough road waiting for my hysterectomy. Because I was in the post-partum period after giving birth, I had not started my monthly periods yet, but the doctors wanted to take every precaution. Finally, I was given monthly injections of Depo Provera. This medication would affect the pituitary gland responsible for ovulation. By having the injections it gave my body a false sense of pregnancy. This was to prevent my body from producing certain hormones to prevent menstruation. By not ovulating and having a period the growth of endometriosis was slowed or possibly stopped. Having the injections meant my menstrual periods would not begin, which also stopped the horrible pain caused by the endometriosis. This gave me additional time to heal from the pregnancy and build up the iron in my blood so that I would be better prepared for surgery.

As it was, I only made it three and a half months before having the surgery rather than the six months waiting period originally planned. I still had abdominal pain; it was just not as severe as in the past. I had a complete hysterectomy, which is a last resort for severe endometriosis. That is because it is major abdominal surgery. The doctor removed the uterus, ovaries, cervix, and fallopian tubes and scraped out the endometriosis for over three and a half hours. I was told there had been tremendous damage and scar tissue. He also informed me he felt confident he removed all the endometriosis but could not give me a one hundred percent guarantee. At the age of 24, I had two children and my childbearing years were officially over. It had been a long road since starting my periods at age eleven and a half.

There was a six-week recovery period and we still had the help of a babysitter since I could not even lift the baby. I was on Coumadin for eight weeks to prevent any blood clots, which required weekly blood tests to check the clotting time.

However, I soon learned the surgery was over but not the battle. I was placed on Premarin as a treatment for menopausal symptoms. It was a hormone replacement prescribed for estrogen deficiency. However the estrogen-related migraines were back. They were as bad if not worse, requiring Demerol shots. After six months I was switched to Ogen, another form of female hormone replacement therapy that was not as intense as Premarin, but the doctor had to keep lowering the dosage. Finally, after a year of horrible headaches they gave up all together. I was not taking estrogen supplements of any kind. I went through the intense hot flashes for about six months waking up in the night totally drenched. I took more cold baths than I could count during that time. Eventually, the hot flashes ended and I went on with my life as a wife and mother. Unfortunately, the headaches continued and so did the treatments for them. After what I had been through, I considered this livable. But still, I was on a dead-end road to osteoporosis and did not know it. If only I had known then what I know now, but hindsight is twenty-twenty. And even if I had known, I'm not sure what my options would have been considering my medical history and intolerance to medications. Additionally, no one mentioned the importance calcium and vitamin D, especially since I was not able to tolerate hormone supplements. I could only assume they did not know then the repercussions to follow later.

Female Reproduction System Prior to the Hysterectomy[10]

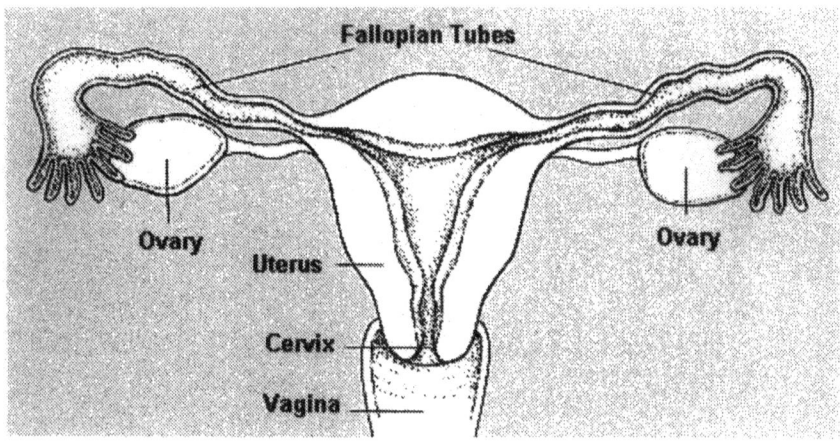

Total Hysterectomy: removes all that is in the circle below.[11]

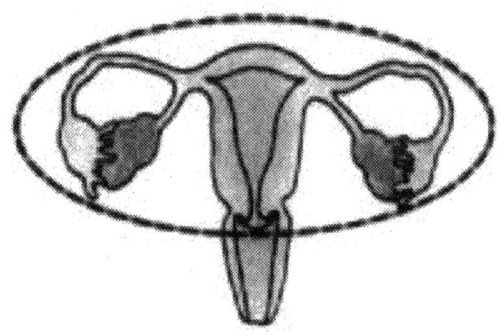

[10, 11] Diagrams courtesy of Lee J. Monlezun, Jr. M.D. FACOG

Chapter 4

In 1985, we were living in Cottonwood, Arizona, when I fell trying to kill a fly. I had broken my right wrist and at the time we thought my back was broken too. My oldest daughter calmly called the operator as I lay on the floor in pain. The police arrived before the ambulance and the officer managed to get inside of the house. Then he met my dog, a Rhodesian Ridgeback who had lived at the Navajo Army Depot in Belmont, Arizona. He had been trained for weaponry and gunpowder prior to becoming my pet. Because the officer was wearing a gun and bullet belt the dog pinned the officer to the wall. I had learned years earlier that a well-trained dog would obey a command from someone other than his owner. So I had converted all his commands into French. I was lying on the floor yelling in French to the dog and the officer kept yelling for me to calm down. When I explained to the officer about the French commands he said to keep yelling at the dog. However, the dog knew I was in danger and he was hesitant to give up. When the ambulance and fire department arrived on the scene they had to wait outside until the animal control officer arrived. The animal control officer finally had to shoot a tranquilizing dart into the dog. Once the dog was sedated the medics were able to come in and treat me.

I was placed in a full cervical spine immobilization as a precaution because of any potential neck injury. The head and neck had to be im-mobilized to reduce movement and keep the head and neck in a neutral alignment. This was a two-man job and as one medic held my head in place with his fingers against my neck and under the corners of my jaw, another applied the rigid one-piece cervical spine immobilization collar. He slid the collar behind my head, sliding the front portion upward until it was around my neck and secured it with a snug fit us-ing Velcro straps.

Since a cervical spine immobilization should not be used alone for spinal immobilization, my body was picked up in a strategic manner and I was carefully placed on a backboard with the assistance of several more medics. I was then strapped to the backboard and duct tape was used to secure the cervical collar to the backboard. They had also im-mobilized the fractured right wrist. By the time they were finished I could not move any part of my body except for my fingers and toes.

After patching into the hospital, they started an intravenous line and gave me pain medication. Once I arrived at the hospital many x-rays were done of my head, neck, spine, and wrist. I had sprained my back badly and had a broken wrist. The wrist was broken on both sides but the fracture had not completely gone through meeting in the middle. My right wrist fracture was known as a "Colles Fracture." which is a wrist fracture involving a break of the end of the radius bone of the forearm ("distal radius fracture"). Most of these fractures occur when an individual attempts to break a fall with their hand. Your body weight can cause a fracture just above the wrist as a result of the impact when you hit the ground. This is also a very common fracture in elderly patients and patients with osteoporosis.

An orthopedic doctor came in and put several injections into my wrist. Then he set it. Oh, my God! Talk about pain! That was worse than initially breaking it. Once it was set (in the most peculiar position) I was allowed to go home. I was given a prescription of strong pain medication, told not to touch the wrist, get it wet, or remove any of the bandaging or stabilizer.

For eight weeks I had regular follow-ups with the doctor. Once the wrist was healed I was surprised there was little therapy that needed to be done. Mostly I had to squeeze a ball with the wrist in certain positions.

Full Cervical Spinal Stabilization

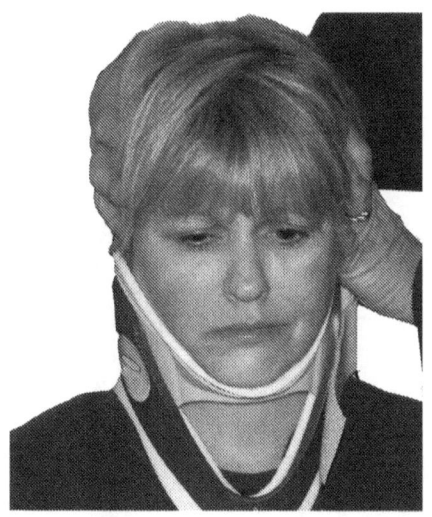

Secured on a Backboard for Transport

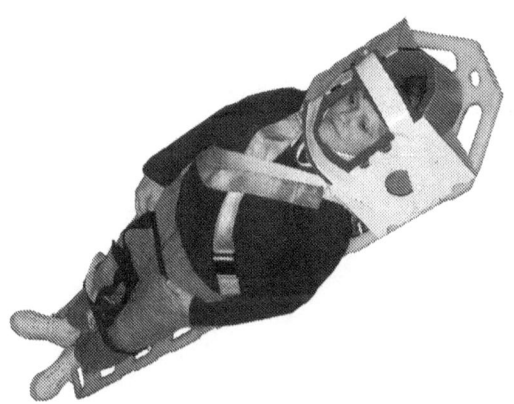

Colles Fracture[12]

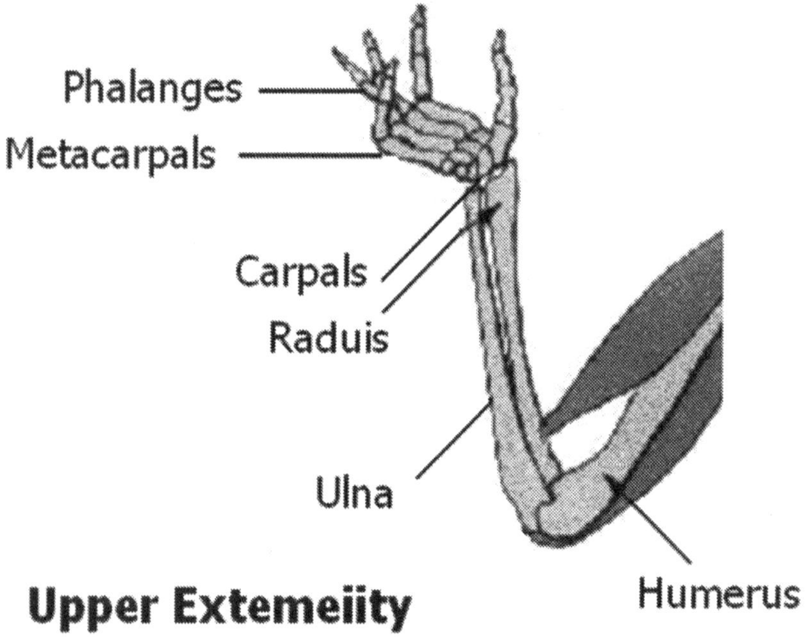

Phalanges

Metacarpals

Carpals

Raduis

Ulna

Humerus

Upper Extemeiity

[12] Photo courtesy of wikipedia.org

Chapter 5

Between the years of 1986 through 1989 we lived in Williams, Arizona, in a two-story Victorian house with a spiral staircase. While living there I broke ribs quite often — sometimes two or three at a time. I broke ribs coughing, sneezing too hard, or as I leaned over the bathtub to scrub. It didn't seem to matter what I did — I just always had broken ribs. Each time it happened I went to the doctor, had x-rays for confirmation of the break, and was given a Velcro wrap to wear. I was averaging between 10-20 rib fractures a year. The amount of broken ribs quickly added up. Because there were so many the doctor kept asking me if my husband was abusing me. I always answered, "No." At this time, I still didn't know I had osteoporosis. I didn't understand the disease enough to pick up the obvious warning signs. And apparently the small town doctor was not seeing the signs either.

Unfortunately with the rib fractures there was not much that could be done to make me more comfortable, except for using a Velcro wrap. Chest x-rays confirmed the fractures and sometimes my doctor requested additional x-rays during the healing process to determine how well I was healing. At times, however, a person can have fractured ribs that would not show up on x-rays.

With a rib fracture there is pain each time you take a deep breath, cough, sneeze, or press over the injured area. There is also pain when you get out of a chair or try to lie down in bed or get up from a night's sleep. For me, certain body movements were definitely limited while healing. There was to be no strenuous activity and any exercise or movement was to be "as tolerated." Ice packs or heat over the injured area was often recommended, but the only thing that truly controlled the discomfort was a prescribed pain medication. Each time I broke ribs the doctor stressed the importance of deep breathing and coughing exercises to prevent lung infections. Using a pillow supported the injured area and helped a little. That exercise, however, was definitely not fun. The doctor also said if I experienced worse pain, a fever of over 101º F, difficulty breathing, abdominal pain, or vomiting, that I should call his office. Fortunately, none of those symptoms ever occurred.

With each fracture I expected an 8-week recovery period. But just as the broken ribs seemed to heal, more would break and the cycle just continued on and on. Because of this I really tried to control the pain medication or it would have been never-ending.

In April of 1988, my husband at that time was working very late one night. Around 11:00 I was going down the spiral staircase, fell, and broke my right leg. Both of our daughters were asleep in their bedrooms located downstairs. I was unable to get up and yelled for approximately ten minutes before my oldest daughter woke up as a result of my yelling. I told her to call her father at work and tell him that I had broken my leg and could not get up. I had also been carrying a glass of water, which had shattered on the hard wood floor. My husband came home, called our local small town doctor and a neighbor lady who lived across the street. She came to stay with the girls and between her and my husband they managed to get me in the backseat of my car.

Once we arrived at the doctor's office, there was a wheelchair to transport me from the car to the inside and x-rays were taken. I had broken the fibula, which is the long thin bone behind the tibia (the large weight-bearing bone). Fortunately, the fracture had not penetrated through the skin and was a closed fracture, so I did not require surgery. Surgery would have added more complications since it would have required an ambulance ride to Flagstaff, 35 miles east of Williams on Interstate 40, plus surgery and recovery. The broken bone was manipulated back in to place (after pain medication had been given and taken affect), and the leg was placed in a steel reinforced immobilizer that was fastened with Velcro.

Luckily, none of my breaks had required a plaster cast. I did need to use crutches and had a very hard time with them. Since the house was two-story with a spiral staircase, I spent the first few days and nights downstairs in my oldest daughter's twin bed. When I was able to finally work my way upstairs I did it sitting down on each step as I went up or down. You can be sure I made those trips as few as possible and had the girls do the running when they were home.

After eight weeks, and reviewing x-rays, the leg was considered healed. I still had to use crutches for a while as I learned to build up the strength in the leg. Since this was my first "major fracture" I was not aware of physical therapy nor did the doctor suggest it. I do remember I felt faint the first time I tried to put full weight on the leg and was grateful for the crutches since the leg did not function well. After approximately a week of the crutches I was able to limp unassisted and eventually gained full use of the right leg.

Crutches for Mobility

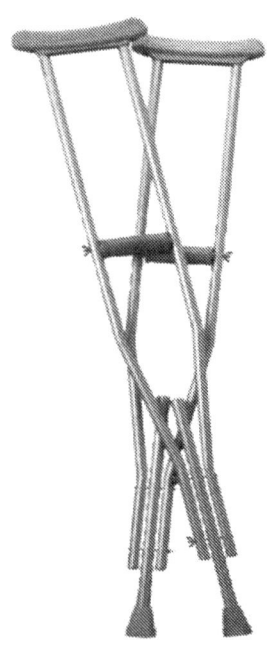

Along with continuous rib fractures, I still experienced violent migraines. So the option of starting an estrogen supplement program still remained out of the question. Then, in late 1989, we moved back to Cottonwood, Arizona. I was desperate to find relief for my painful migraines. In May 1991, my family internist in Sedona, Arizona, suggested a physical therapist that had success treating migraine patients. He used a technique where the patient was strapped by the chin to a door (as I recall). However, before he treated a patient he always did neck and spine x-rays. He came back into my room with the x-rays stating he would not touch me with a ten-foot pole. I had bad osteoporosis, needed to see my family internist, and he suggested getting a referral to the Mayo Clinic in Scottsdale, Arizona. He also knew about my fractures from filling out new patient forms. The rib fractures were averaging a good twenty plus a year at this time.

I was stunned to say the least. I always had lower back pain, but I attributed that to previous falls. I had broken my right wrist and right leg, but again I blamed those on falls. I had the ever-constant rib fractures, which I could not explain. I seemed to fall a lot but could not explain why except for the fact my right leg gave out. Except for the migraines and broken bones, when it came to any other pain, I was able to tolerate it. Still, I was too unfamiliar with osteoporosis so the warning signs were not flashing in neon.

After hearing this news I immediately saw my doctor who referred me to the Mayo Clinic. To say I was in for a big shock is an understatement. I was only 35; how could this have happened? It simply could not have been true. It had to be a mistake. I went into instant denial. This was something that was to affect older people, not me.

It was hard to believe that I had osteoporosis at the age of 35. Unfortunately, I had not known or recognized the signs. Despite having had broken ribs, a wrist, and a leg, my husband, parents, and I had all remained clueless until now—probably because I was so young. I knew osteoporosis was a loss of calcium to the bone. I knew about the stooped posture because my mother had it. But I did not understand all the mechanics involved; what caused it and its consequences, how we could fix it or what changes would have to be made in my lifestyle. Deep down I hoped that once I met with the doctor at the Mayo Clinic I would be told that was not it. Instead of osteoporosis I had something else. What that would be never crossed my mind; I was just trying to deny it. I also had no idea what type of tests were involved. Would they be painful? No one in the medical field gave me any explanations of what to expect or how the problem would be fixed. All I could do was to continue to wait patiently for my scheduled appointment on June 18, 1991, and that was six weeks away.

Chapter 6

Finally, the day arrived and my husband and mother went with me for my first appointment to the Mayo Clinic in Scottsdale, Arizona. To say I was terrified was an understatement. I didn't know what to expect, what tests would be performed, or if the tests would be painful. I had a lot of questions for the doctor: How did this happen? What could be done to fix it? How long would it take to fix?

The Mayo Clinic was a very impressive building. A concierge held open the door and greeted us as we walked in. The entire staff was well dressed, soft-spoken, and extremely polite. They made me feel as if I was the only patient and that their main purpose was to assist me. They could not have been more gracious and comforting. As I pre-registered and went to various departments for different tests, a representative was with me the entire time until I was taken to my doctor's office.

I was informed a normal x-ray was not sufficient enough to measure bone density. It could, however, show spinal fractures, damaged discs, and explain the cause of height loss if applicable. To determine if someone had osteoporosis a bone mineral density (BMD) test could be performed, which measures the amount of calcium in the bones with emphasis on areas such as a leg, a hip, and the spinal column.

"Dual Energy X-ray Absorptiometry," or DXA, is one of the most accurate and precise forms of a BMD test, detecting as little as 1% change in the bone mass. It measures the amount of bone loss and the degree of osteoporosis and can estimate if the patient will be at risk if they do not already have osteoporosis. The results are then reported as a "T" score and "Z" score. The "T" score compares the bone density to a 30 year old (the age when a person reaches their peak bone mass). The "Z" score compares the bone mass density to a healthy person of the same age and ethnic background as the person who was tested.

This test can be done as an outpatient and the scanning takes only a few minutes. Registration takes longer than the actual testing. No fasting, medication, or advance preparation is needed. In fact, you don't even need to change out of your street clothes unless your clothing has metal buttons, buckles, or zippers. You only need to remove any jewelry being worn at the time. It is completely painless and only takes about ten to twenty minutes. You just lay very still on an x-ray table while a machine scans certain parts of your body (the leg, hip, spine, and/or total body; most major fractures are in these locations). In a couple of days your doctor will have the results. For people who are concerned about radiation exposure, the dose is about one-tenth of what a chest x-ray is.

BMD testing is recommended for postmenopausal women (especially if they have experienced fractures); younger women who are postmenopausal (because of a hysterectomy) with risk factors for osteoporosis; women with increased risk for the disease; and women over the age of 50. It is also important to do a follow-up every year thereafter, especially if there is a history of fractures.

Some doctors ask for a urine test also, which may indicate bone loss as well from the amount of collagen found in testing the urine sample. Ultrasound and CT scanning are other ways of testing, but DXA is the preferred by most doctors.

All kinds of tests were performed on me, including the DXA to measure my bone mineral density. An electrocardiogram (ECG) was the first test that was done (to check my heart). They also took urine samples and recorded my height and weight. They did have trouble drawing my blood, but that was quite common for me. A number of x-rays were also taken. The drawing of blood was the only uncomfortable procedure.

All I had to do was wait to meet the doctor and hear the verdict. I was still in denial and quite confident he would say I had something else — just not osteoporosis. After all, I was only 35 years old, a wife, and mother of two young daughters. This was not supposed to happen to me. It might happen to somebody else but not me. Little did I know that what I was about to hear would change my life forever.

When I first met my doctor at the Mayo Clinic, an endocrinologist, he introduced himself to my mother thinking she was the patient. He was absolutely stunned to find out it was me. He had looked at the tests results but not really at the age of the patient he was reading about. I was already scared going in and now I was terrified because of his reaction. I had no clue how important and devastating his next words were going to be. The doctor explained that osteoporosis, which means "porous bones," is a painless disease until the bones become so weak or brittle that they begin to break. Some people refer to it as a "silent disease."

It is caused by a loss of calcium, phosphorus and minerals necessary for the bones to remain strong. When the strength of those bones is weakened, there will be a loss of that calcium, phosphorus, and minerals. A drop in estrogen levels also contributes to the cause of osteoporosis. Vitamin D is essential for the absorption of calcium. An inadequate amount will accelerate the bone loss process even if you are taking calcium.

Throughout our life bone, a living, active tissue is changing within us. New bone is constantly being made (by cells called osteoblasts) as old bone is broken down (by cells called ostoeclasts). And when we are younger we build new bone at a faster rate than it is broken down. However as we get older, and after reaching our bone mass peak, we continue to build bone but at a slower rate, losing more than we build. At around age 30, the maximum bone mass has achieved its peak density. Then it starts to lose mass. Heredity can also be an influence in pre-determining if someone is more likely to become a victim to osteoporosis. The risk factor rises for daughters if their mother had a history of bone loss or fractures.

Suddenly you break a rib and all you did was sneeze too hard. You begin to experience lower back pain. In more severe cases patients can experience loss of height and spinal deformities (like a stooped posture) and repeated fractures.

Depending on the type of fracture, major surgery and hospitalization may be necessary. After weeks or months of healing, it can be followed by even more months of physical therapy with no guarantee for a one hundred percent recovery. It is discouraging knowing there are more fractures to come as the years go by. For some, mobility can become so restricted that the use of a cane, crutches, walker, wheelchair, or scooter may be required.

It's hard to be careful when you don't feel the affects of osteoporosis. You don't realize the precautions that are necessary. When there is no injury, you are not familiar with the signs and symptoms. It's also easy to forget and continue with your normal daily routine. But when you break a bone or hurt yourself you are careful and favor the injury. When you are suffering from an injury or serious fracture, reality quickly meets you head on. Early detection is important in slowing down the process of osteoporosis.

I was told I had severe osteoporosis, which was considered serious, especially for my age. I was 35 with the bones of an 80 year old. An x-ray of the lumbar spine showed mild hypertrophic (nourishment) changes and degenerative changes. A thoracic spine x-ray revealed evidence of demineralization as well as hypertrophic changes.

At this time in 1991, the doctor told me my bone mineral density tests results were as follows:

My bone mineral density for the lumbar spine (L2-4) was $0.714g/cm^2$. The bone mineral density was only 67% of what was normal adjusted for my age and sex. This was below the fracture threshold of $0.83g/cm^2$. The lumbar vertebral bone density was more than two standard deviations below normal again adjusted for my age and sex. The bone mineral density of my left femoral neck region was $0.668g/cm^2$. This bone mineral density was 77% of what was normal adjusted for my age and sex. The femoral neck density was within two standard deviations of normal after adjustment for the age and sex.

- T SPINE (Thoracic Spine)

  There was demineralization of the thoracic spine and hypo plastic 12th ribs.

- L SPINE (Lumbar Spine)

  There were minimal hypertrophic changes to the lumbar spine and mild degenerative changes in the lower lumbar facet joints. Old rib fractures were also evident.

The doctor explained that my premature menopause was a significant contributor to the osteoporosis, and the fact that I had not been taking estrogen replacement (hormone replacement therapy also known as HRT), for all those years was a big factor. I asked why nobody told me back in 1980 what would happen without estrogen supplements. His reply was that back then they didn't know. Even if they had known, I had the complication of migraines when I did take estrogen supplements. Over the years, new studies produce new findings and at the time of my hysterectomy it just was not known. I had shrunk one half of an inch in height and I was only five foot two to begin with. The doctor also asked if we had children. When I responded that we had two daughters he said they would be at risk in their later years because of the family history with osteoporosis.

A good way to explain osteoporosis is to think of a savings account. Each time you are ovulating you are building up calcium in the bone. If the normal woman has a natural menopause that may begin in the late forties or early fifties (some start earlier or later), she is building up that saving account. When she finally reaches menopause and is no longer ovulating, the savings account is no longer building up. Once a woman has reached her bone mass peak she begins to lose more bone than she builds back up. That is when she begins to use up that savings account. By the time women are in the sixties, seventies, or eighties, depending on the individual, the savings account is virtually empty. This results in osteoporosis — the lack of calcium in the bone and the deterioration of bone tissue.

In my case I never had a chance to build up that savings account. So it depleted quickly with osteoporosis resulting at a young age. Estrogen replacement had been aborted because of the complications with my migraines. Calcium intake was virtually non-existent since I had been taken off of most milk products when I was around 11 years old because of allergies. I know my mother and maternal grandmother had osteoporosis. My grandmother had even experienced hip fractures. My mother, grandmother, and maternal great-grandmother all had the stooped posture. My mother even had to buy blouses and dresses a size larger than needed in order to accommodate the hump on her back. With all this family history, I was doomed from the start.

I was told not to lift anything over ten pounds in weight. That just yanking the sheets really hard while making the bed was enough to break my neck. At any given time there would probably be a thousand hairline cracks to the spine. I was also told that I needed to swim every day for the rest of my life since the buoyancy of water would protect the bones during exercise. Mild weight bearing exercise was also suggested. Exercising helps build strong bones and slows down bone loss. The earlier in life you start the better. But you can start at any age. I was no longer able to go horseback riding. This was something I absolutely loved but didn't get to do often; now I couldn't do it at all. Long periods of bending and stooping were also not recommended because of the weakness to my spine. The doctor told me that by the time I was 45 years old, I will have had complete hip replacement in both hips.

Finally, the doctor said he was going to start me on a calcium supplement treatment. I would start receiving Calcimar injections shortly after returning home. Hopefully this medicine would help prevent further bone loss. There was nothing to build bone back up, just medication to prevent further loss. My internist in Sedona would oversee the treatments since I didn't live in the Phoenix/ Scottsdale area. In addition, I would need to begin taking on a daily basis one thousand milligrams of calcium (pill form: 500 in the morning and 500 in the evening) and Vitamin D. Vitamin D was essential for calcium and phosphorus metabolism.

All of this information was extremely overwhelming and sobering. My husband and mother were in as much shock as I was. But I do remembering telling the doctor I was bound and determined to still have my own hips at 45. The thought of that made me feel weak. Having experienced broken bones I knew I did not want to go there. Plus, I remembered my mother's stories about my grandmother's recoveries from hip surgeries.

There was certainly a lot to digest from all that the doctor had told us. It was a somber two-hour drive home from Phoenix. My husband and I also had to discuss how we were going to tell our daughters. Many lifestyle changes were going to affect the entire family as we implemented the new restrictions placed on me.

Bone Mineral Density Machine

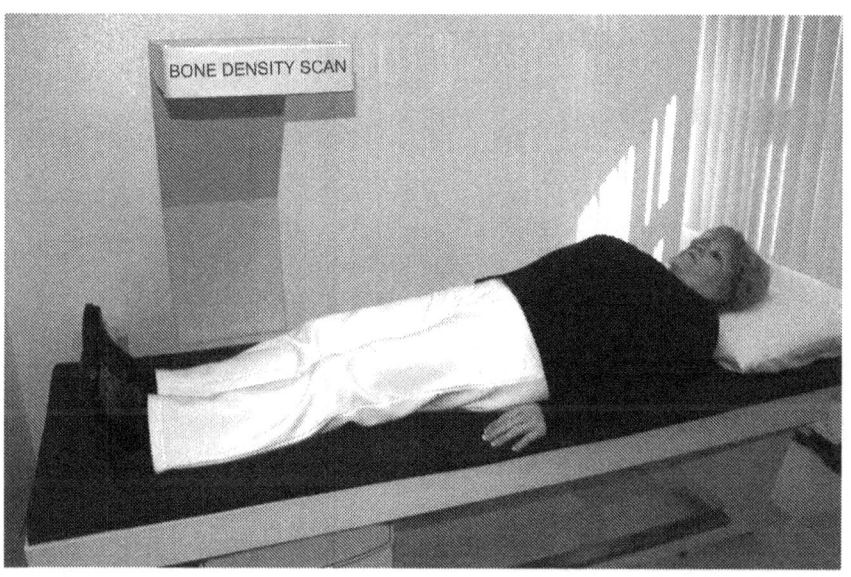

A Bone Mineral Density (BMD) test is painless and takes approximately ten minutes.

Chapter 7

Once we were back home, my husband and I sat down with our two daughters. The girls were all too familiar with my continuing saga of broken bones and had been frightened by it, so they were quite anxious to hear about the meeting with the doctor.

As simply as possible, we explained to them what osteoporosis was. We said it was a loss of calcium to the bones that made bones thinner and weaker. That was why I kept breaking bones, especially ribs, so easily. When they asked how I got it we tried to explain the causes of the disease and that I had most of those causes: the premature hysterectomy, no hormone replacement therapy, small boned body structure, no supplemental calcium intake, Caucasian race, and family history (their maternal grandmother and their great-grandmother had had it). Osteoporosis was something I was bound to get no matter what. Too many factors were against me.

We explained about the hairline cracks in my spine and how easily I could break my neck if I was not careful. At that time we also explained the new limitations placed on me. They would have to help me more since I had a limit of lifting no more than ten pounds (that was equal to a sack of potatoes). Every time I had broken a leg or wrist the girls had always been very helpful so I knew they would be supportive of these changes. Gardening was a passion for me, but bending and stooping to weed and plant was something that I would need to change. My younger daughter suggested a stool to sit on. I also told them that they would have to help pick the produce from our summer and winter gardens since the full basket would quickly exceed ten pounds. If I did fall, I had to be very careful about getting up. It could make the difference in never walking again.

There was quite a bit of excitement when we told the girls that we would be getting a swimming pool larger than the one we already had. We already had a small above ground pool that was eighteen feet in diameter, but the doctor had told me I had to swim everyday. What we already had would not be efficient enough for vigorous laps.

The girls were told I would begin medical treatments to hopefully prevent any further bone loss. There was a medication called Calcimar that had to be given by injection at the doctor's office. It did not build bone back up but could help reduce future loss. Hopefully I would be able to tolerate the medication since I had a history of intolerance.

After all the news had been told, both girls cried but understood what was going on. They just kept asking why it had to be me. Then they wanted to know if they would get it and when since I had it so young. I explained to them that there was a very good chance of them getting osteoporosis when they were older because of all the family medical history. But if they did all the right things now and throughout their lives they would probably be much, much older then me when it happened. They needed to get good exercise, plenty of calcium, and vitamin D and if they ever had to have a hysterectomy (endometriosis can be hereditary), to take hormone replacement therapy.

At least they understood why I periodically had broken bones. There was now an answer to the cause. With that understanding maybe the new changes would be easier to accept and implement.

Chapter 8

Treatment is essential in preventing and/or slowing down the osteoporosis process. It's important for the patient to meet with their personal doctor who will prescribe the best course of action depending on the patient's medical history. Unlike when I was diagnosed, there are many options available today for helping osteoporosis, but there is always the chance of serious side effects and health risks depending on the medication and the patient. The doctor needs to monitor the patient's treatment closely.

This was something I was to learn firsthand. Once back home I went to the Sedona Medical Center and met with my family internist where I began the treatment of Calcimar injections. The treatment lasted about two months before it was decided I truly could not tolerate the medication. I had terrible vomiting, and horrible intestinal discomfort. So we were back to square one. As new drugs were expected to come out we would start another treatment as soon as we could.

A certain health condition may require the use of a vitamin above the usual recommended daily allowance. I was also informed it was necessary to take vitamin D when taking a calcium supplement. Vitamin D is essential for absorbing the calcium and phosphorus that is required for the normal development of bones (and teeth). As I mentioned earlier, my doctor recommended the appropriate dosage for me based on my weight and after considering the other medications being taken on a daily basis.

How a patient accepts and responds to new lifestyle changes can determine the outcome of their mobility later in life. It's vital that they embrace the changes. It is also very important that the entire family of the patient understands the disease, the necessary changes in lifestyle, and that they are supportive and helpful of those restrictions. It requires a commitment from everyone because it affects everyone, not just the person with the disease.

Regular exercise was and still is a necessary ingredient for helping the bones. We bought a new above ground pool. It was the largest one Doughboy made at the time — it was truly huge. We lived on over an acre of land so we had plenty of room for it. It took a week for the business we bought it from to prepare the ground, assemble and fill the pool. Living in Arizona made the swimming season last pretty long and I tried to be faithful about it. It also guaranteed me a great tan. The swimming definitely seemed to make a difference. I was still breaking ribs, but not as often.

Walking is a healthy weight-bearing exercise that was also pre-scribed. I began walking around in my cul-de-sac three to four times a week. I often, however, felt a lot of lower back pain afterwards. I continued to walk anyway because of the importance in building strength in both the muscles and the bones. Walking became easier after I invested in a treadmill, which allowed me to walk at any time without worrying about the weather— whether it was too hot in the summer or cool in the winter. By walking shorter amounts several times a day I did not suffer as much lower back pain.

I also had to learn to move slower (I was always walking fast, work-ing fast etc), watch what I lifted since I had a ten pound restriction, try not to cough or sneeze too hard, and just basically restructure my entire life to be more cautious. If I fell I was to get medical help. The chances that my spine may be more injured than I thought were high. It could mean the difference in ever walking again.

These new lifestyle changes were a lot harder than one can imagine. As hard as I tried to abide by the new daily restrictions, I did have trouble sticking to the rules. I have to be honest and say I absolutely hate taking pills. Calcium pills seemed to be so large (horse pills by my standards). I did and still do have trouble taking them. Eventually I found liquid calcium that did not taste bad and I was able to commit to taking it daily.

By doing exactly what I was told to do and not do meant this whole disease was real. I was still trying to deny it— both to myself and to others. I did not want the appearance of being "handicapped." There was also a part of me that did not even think about it when doing things I should not do. After all I had a regular routine that I had followed for so many years. How many people actually consider how much a six-pack of pop weighs (almost five pounds) when shopping at the grocery store, or many other items for that matter?

I found it also hard to sit on a stool to do my gardening. I was constantly getting up and down, so, I continued to stoop, and at night I certainly felt the pain from it. The yards did continue to remain beautiful and flourished, but I definitely did pay a physically painful price for it.

When I did fall, we learned to call 911. I would then be transported by ambulance with full c-spine precautions to our local hospital. Once x-rays showed no spinal or neck damages, the backboard and paraphernalia were removed and finally I would be allowed to return home. Unfortunately, our local fire department got to know me very well. They were aware my situation and were always very kind.

It's like I had mentioned earlier in the book, when you don't hurt it's hard to remember you can no longer do something. And since denial plays a major role, you tell yourself it can't be true. Then you realize both how true and bad it is once you break the next bone.

Treadmill for Weight-bearing Exercise

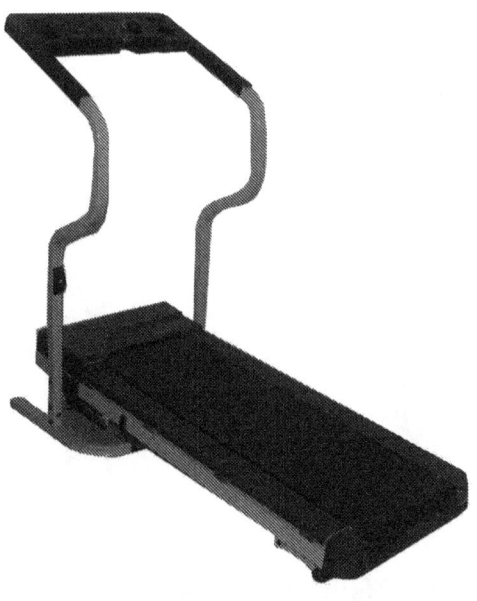

Having my own treadmill gave me the freedom to exercise when I wanted. Despite the weather outdoors, I could remain comfortable whether it was cold in the winter or hot in the summer.

Swimming Pool

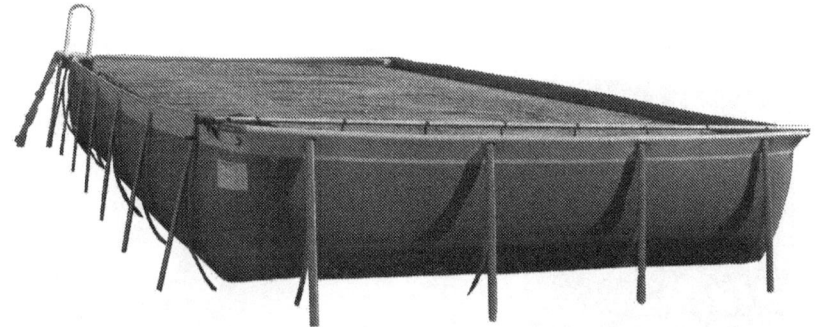

In my case non-weight bearing exercise is crucial and swimming strengthens the muscles while the buoyancy from water protects the bones. Stronger muscles protect the bones from serious trauma.

Do you know what your groceries weigh?

Half-gallon milk?

Fabric Softener?

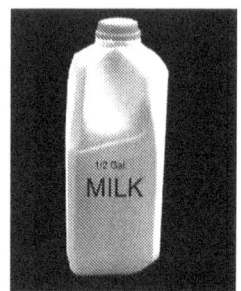

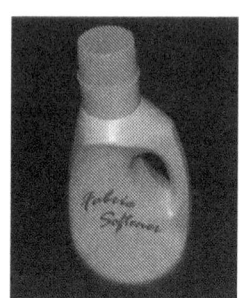

Half-gallon ice cream?

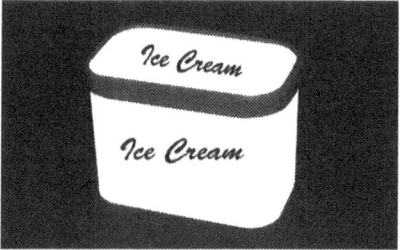

18-Count Eggs?

6-Pack of Soda Pop?

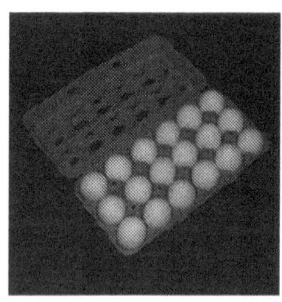

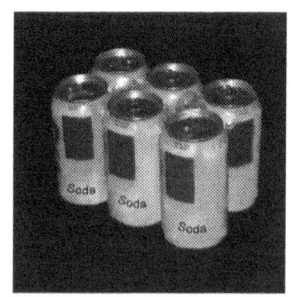

Chapter 9

In September of 1992, I went back to the Mayo Clinic for an annual exam. In the past year I had suffered over thirteen rib fractures with mild trauma. I had also experienced mild back pain, which the doctor said was clearly attributed to the osteoporosis. A new bone density test showed significant drop in bone density since the tests the previous year. I now had a greater bone loss compared to last year's bone loss already on record. There was also an exaggerated lumbar lordosis of the spine (abnormal curve to the front of the spine) with pain in the lumbar area.

Once the doctor came into my examination room, he said I was nothing short of a "therapeutic dilemma" in view of my intolerance to the medications and complications with estrogen replacement therapy because of the migraines. He then suggested treatment with an investigational drug called Didronel. The required dosage was 200mg twice a day for 15 days every three months. Even though the drug was considered investigational, there were no other options available.

He gave me the results of my BMD test which were:

- T SPINE (Thoracic Spine)
  The bone density for the left femoral neck was 0.621g/cm². This bone mineral density was 72% of normal for my age and

sex. And the femoral neck density was more than two standard deviations below normal again for age and sex.

- L SPINE (Lumbar Spine)

  My bone density for the lumbar spine (L 1-3) was $0.683g/cm^2$. This was 68% of normal adjusted for my age and sex. This was below the fracture threshold of $0.83g/cm^2$. The lumbar vertebral bone density was more than two standard deviations below normal, again adjusted for my age and sex.

The doctor informed me I was not to sit too long, stand too long, or anything else. The purpose was to not put so much weight or pressure on the lower back. The use of a reclining chair was ordered to distribute the weight to help prevent further rib fractures. The doctor even wrote a prescription for my insurance company accompanied by a letter stressing the importance of the recliner. I was to continue walking and swimming. To avoid placing any stress on the back; I was not to lift anything over eight to ten pounds. I couldn't put myself in a position that could cause sudden stress to the hip or spine area.

Since I had so many rib fractures the past year, the doctor didn't want any more x-rays done because of the exposure to radiation. He said I knew when a rib was broken, and that I should call and tell my local doctor when and how it happened. I needed to be very conservative in my activities and take every precaution to protect my back.

Over the years we tried other medications for osteoporosis. Fosamax, Evista, and nasal therapy with Calcitonin were other medications for calcium therapy that were tried and failed because of adverse reactions. Many of those medications were still considered investigative, but I had no other options to lean towards. I was also taking over the counter calcium supplements and experiencing severe intestinal problems.

Discouragement was high on the list. It was easy to feel like there was no point in trying because nothing seemed to work. My bones continued to deteriorate regardless of the restrictions placed on me. The medicines were physically intolerable. I saw no hope or light at the end of the tunnel. I started to have the "I don't care attitude" which lasted only until the next broken rib (not too long). Then I had a quick reality dose slapping me back in shape.

Despite my discouragement, I continued to try and be careful and follow the rules. This included the large calcium pills. We purchased a recliner chair like the doctor suggested and I used it regularly. Walking and swimming remained high on the list for physical activity. I still did my gardening, but my daughters helped me out a lot. Usually one of them went with me to the grocery store to help with lifting. Life seemed to go on until the next major fracture.

Recliner Chair

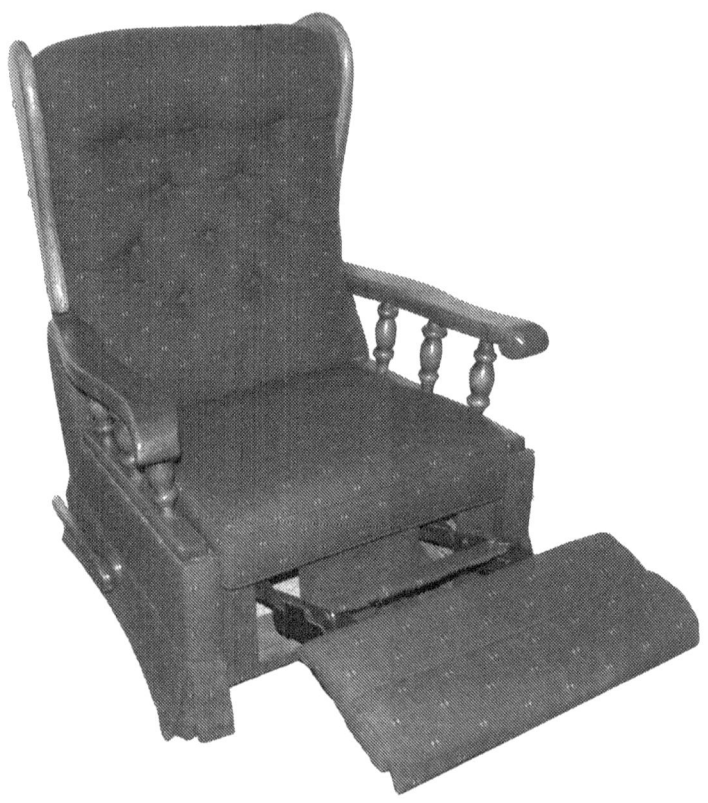

I use a reclining chair for even weight distribution when reading and watching television.

Chapter 10

1993 was not a very good year. In early August, everyone had gone to bed except for me. I had been watching late night television. Around 11:30, as I got up from the recliner, I fell and broke my left wrist and a couple of ribs. I remember standing there and wondering if the wrist was really broken. I tried to twist and turn it just to be sure. Yes, it was definitely broken and the pain had started to kick in. I already knew for certain the ribs were broken. So I went and woke up my husband. I told him I broke my wrist and that we needed to go to the hospital emergency room.

Once at the emergency room I was given an injection for the pain since the fracture was obvious. X-rays were then taken of my wrist. The ribs were not x-rayed, but a Velcro wrap was put on me for the ribs. I really didn't like to wear it and rarely did at home. Since I was short (five feet and one and a half inches) the Velcro wrap was very uncomfortable. It was always cutting in to me just below my breasts making the area raw. I was, and still am, very large breasted (thanks to my paternal grandmother), so the wrap cutting in was just plain miserable- almost as much as the broken ribs. It just seemed easier to hold my ribs when coughing or sneezing instead of wearing that Velcro.

The hardest movement with broken ribs was and still is getting in and out of bed. I would grab the top sheet and inch my way up or down. Getting out of the bathtub proves just as difficult, so I usually take showers.

After the left wrist was x-rayed, the doctor came in and said that the x-rays revealed a minimally displaced fracture — less than five degrees. The diagnosis was a left distal radial and ulnar fracture. The distal (end) part of the radius, located on the inside part of the forearm is the larger of the two bones. The ulna found on the outside of the forearm is thinner. Via eight smaller bones in the wrist joint, the two bones connect the forearm to the hand.

In my case the broken edges remained close enough together that simple manipulation realigned the bones involved (known as a reduction of the fracture). If the fracture had been more complex meaning a number of pieces of bone or the joint was involved surgery would have been required. But I was lucky.

The orthopedic doctor recommended a short arm splint (wrist gauntlet 10 ½ inch splint) followed by a sling. I was told the wrist had to be immobilized and protected for a minimum of six weeks or longer. I was allowed to remove the brace and wrap once a day for bathing. There were no guarantees on the extent of recovery, but the usual patient with this type of fracture did fairly well. Due to the osteoporosis, healing time would be longer than it would be for someone without osteoporosis. Around one o'clock in the morning I was given a prescription for pain medication, told not to use the left hand, and was released to go home.

The broken wrist really limited what I could do, especially since I was left- handed. My daughters had to step in and help. I struggled with cooking and could not do the dishes. I needed help making the bed, changing the sheets and gardening. Swimming was totally out at that point. Being left-handed, bathing was a challenge along with doing my hair and makeup. The last time I broke my wrist it was the right one so I still could do a lot. This time I could not even sign a check. The girls got good at doing that for me too. I was able to drive, but did so very cautiously and tried to be aware of everything around me. Karen, my oldest daughter, had just gotten her learner's permit so she did a lot of the driving for me, especially in the beginning when I was on pain medication. One of my best friends', Bobby, who lived next door, drove me around quite a bit too.

Another very good friend of mine, Michelle, was expecting a baby and I had planned on giving her a shower with another friend of hers. Invitations for 50 women had gone out. To say I panicked would have been an understatement. The shower was moved to Michelle's church and my daughters immediately began organizing things. The shower was scheduled for the middle of September so there was plenty of time for changes.

I was also very grateful it was only August because my husband was turning 40 in October, and I was having a surprise party with a sit down dinner for 30 people to celebrate. At least the wrist would be healed and partially mobile by then. So the girls filled out the invitations since I could not write. Then we planned the menu, the type of decorations, etc.

Just because all these plans were in the works didn't mean the wrist wasn't a problem. When I had broken the wrist, like my previous wrist fracture, the bone on either side had broken but the break had not met in the middle. I was in constant pain that was quite intense. For the first several weeks, pain medication was taken on a very regular basis. Fortunately, the break had not required any surgery.

One week after the fracture occurred I had an appointment for a follow-up with the doctor. Two x-rays were taken, showing no significant change in the fracture. There continued to be swelling around the left wrist and I had full finger and thumb motion. Ten times a day I was to do finger flexing exercises. For the next two weeks, x-rays were taken weekly showing no significant change in the fracture. Each time I was told to continue the finger exercises. Throughout the healing process it was important to have exercise therapy. Its purpose was to preserve movement flexibility and build strength. The appropriate treatment recommended by the doctor depended on the location and severity of the fracture.

I later read that according to the National Institute of Health - Osteoporosis and Related Bone Diseases, the wrist is the most common type of fracture before the age of 75. That number increases at menopause and plateaus after age 65, most likely due to the bone loss following menopause. Wrist fractures occur more often in women that are relatively healthy and active and have good reflexes. The most common wrist fractures occurs when extending the arm to break a fall (that is what I did). The hand and forearm takes all the weight and force from the fall, and one of the wrist bones breaks (I broke both bones).

Just five weeks later, during the middle of September, while carrying food to the refrigerator in the garage, I fell down and landed wedged between the refrigerator and the wheel of my van. My husband had been in the garage with me at the time. I told him to call 911 and that I had just broken more ribs and my right kneecap. The Fire Department showed up and could not believe the predicament I was in. But I had protected the broken wrist! After all, the splint was to come off soon.

Using the backboard, they wedged it between the vehicle tire and me so the van could be pulled out of the garage. The medics needed room to work. Once the vehicle was out of the garage I was secured to the backboard with a full c-spine precaution and transported to the hospital again for more x-rays. While en route the medic spoke to the emergency room and told them there was clearly swelling about the inferior pole of the right patella (a bone situated in front of the kneecap) and obvious discoloration. Fortunately, it was a simple fracture meaning it had not broken through the skin.

It was embarrassing to think I was on a first name basis with most of the personnel in the emergency room. But I had no choice each time I fell and everyone knew it. I was given morphine for the pain prior to x-rays. After the x-rays were taken and read the doctor informed me what I already knew; I had fractured the right patella and numerous ribs. No matter how many times I broke a bone, no matter how much medicine they gave, when it came to setting the bone, I just wanted to die. All I could think was how many more times in my life would I have to go through this.

As I waited for my orthopedic doctor to arrive, I just kept thinking my body was one major mess. I had a broken right patella, a broken left wrist, and broken ribs all at the same time. I had just tapered down on the pain pills for the wrist. But with a newly broken kneecap, I was back to taking more pain medication again on a very regular basis. The doctor also told me there was the possibility of cartilage damage that could lead to post-traumatic arthritis. Again, I was very lucky. X-rays revealed the fracture was non- displaced and was treated without surgery. But I had to be extremely careful. I could only use one crutch, not two, because of the wrist. The knee was immobilized, a prescription for stronger pain medicine was given to me, and once again I was sent home. For the first few days I had to use an ice pack intermittently to reduce swelling. If I experienced increased chest pain, cough, fever, or shortness of breath I was to seek medical attention right away.

Not only could I not write, but I also couldn't drive. My oldest daughter definitely got her driving practice in. I was dependent on her for transportation. With help, the baby shower was a success. Everyone thought I was nuts to have even done it in my situation, but it was something I had to do. I needed to feel normal even when I was not.

As I planned my husband's surprise party my parents were very helpful with suggestions. My father drove me to Phoenix on several occasions to check out the things I needed. There was food, beverage, tablecloths, decorations, etc. The theme was an "Over the Hill Party," and once everything was purchased it was hidden at both my parents and neighbor's house until the day of the party.

On the day of the party, my daughters decorated the house and tables, lined the house and street with helium filled balloons and served the food. Knowing my predicament, friends offered to help out. One was the bartender and another passed out hot hors d'oeuvres. I had prepared the food with the girls help. Amazingly my husband was surprised and we pulled it off. All while I had a broken kneecap, ribs, and wrist.

There were regular follow-ups for both major fractures. As the healing process went on physical therapy exercises were also introduced. The exercises were definitely painful, but necessary if I was going to get back as much mobility as possible.

Physical therapy was necessary for both the wrist and leg and could be done from home. For the wrist I had to squeeze a ball and do rotation exercises. The leg required leg lifts using ankle weights.

Eventually all the bones (ribs included) healed and life went back to normal. Chronic pain due to post-traumatic arthritis for the injury should not be a surprise if it happens. I did, and still do experience arthritis, but only when the weather is cold and/or damp. I can always tell when a storm is brewing.

Left distal radial and ulnar fracture[13]

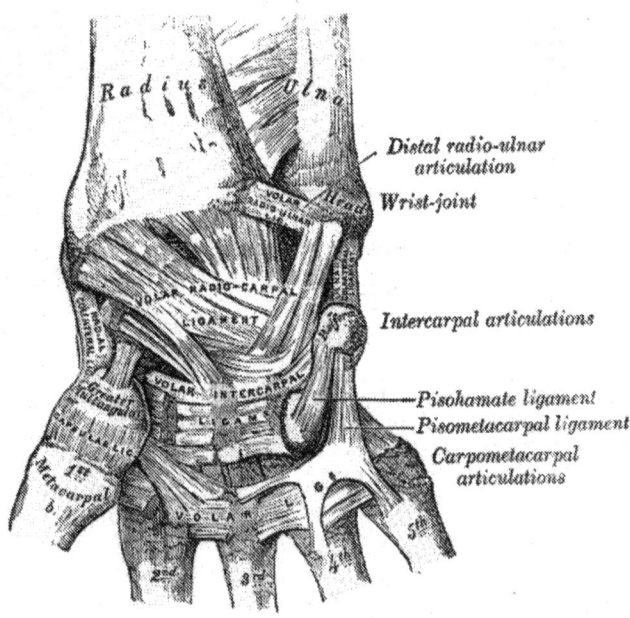

Left distal radial and ulnar fracture Continued[14]

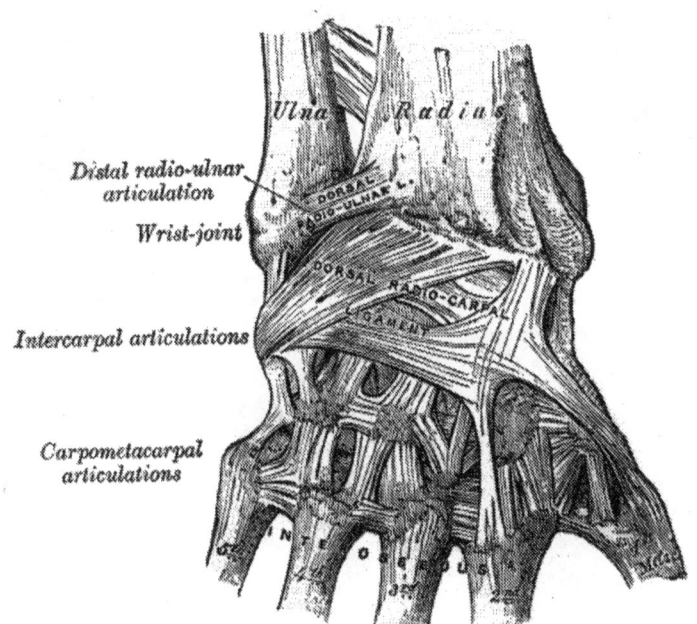

[13, 14] Photo courtesy of wikipedia.org

First I was placed in a full cervical spinal stabilization.

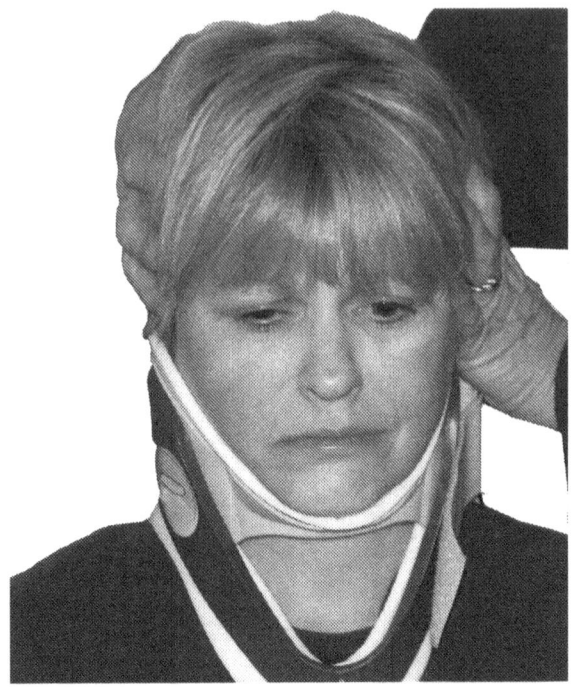

Then, I was secured on a backboard.

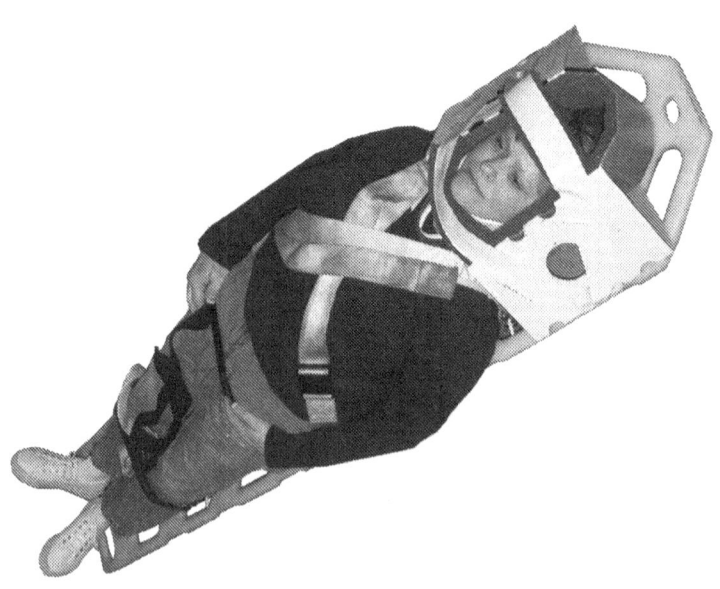

**Then I was transported to the hospital all
because of an osteoporosis injury.**

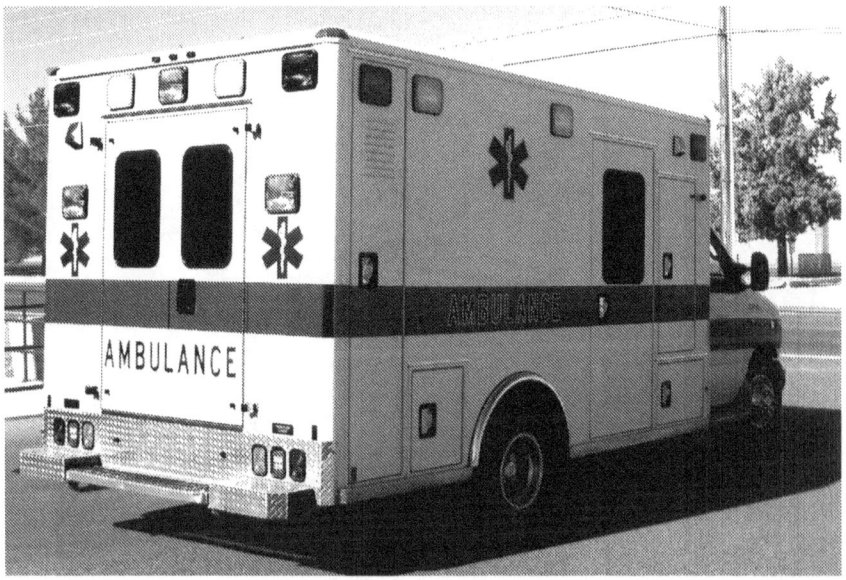

Fractured Right Patella (Kneecap)

Fractured Kneecap

Knee

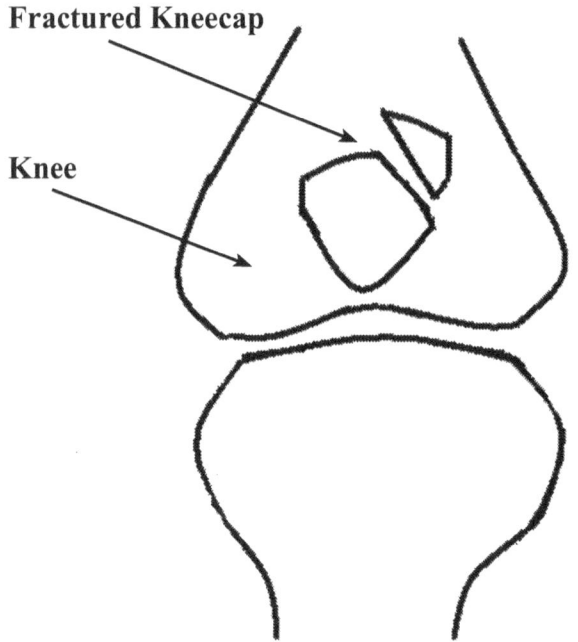

Knee Immobilizer

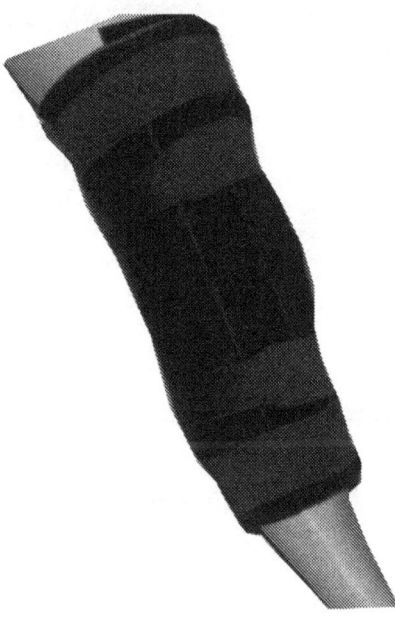

This is a knee stabilizer similar to the one I wore for my fractured right patella.

Physical Therapy For The Right Patella

Straight Leg Exercises

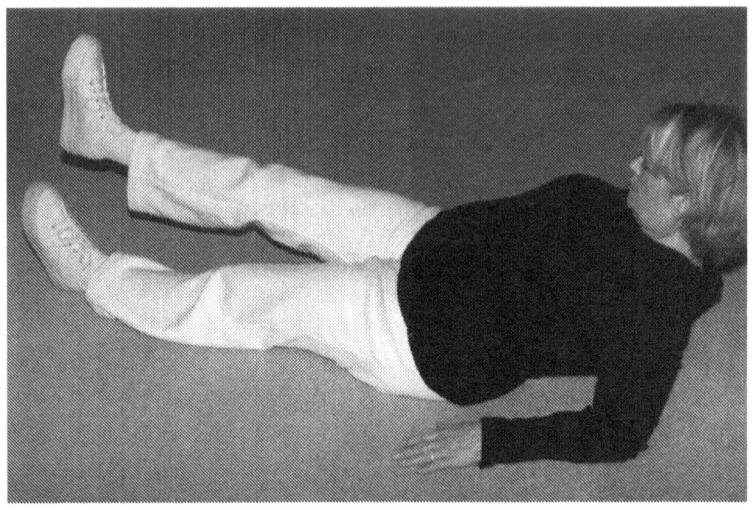

Rest on forearms; tighten muscles on front of thigh
then
lift leg 8-10 inches from surface, keeping knees locked.
Hold for 5 seconds. Repeat 10 times. Do 1 session per day.

Strengthening Exercise

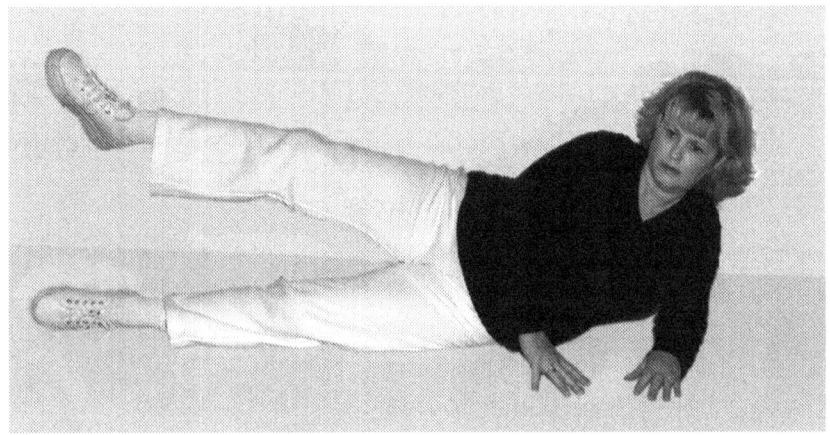

Lying on side, tighten muscles on front of thigh, then lift
leg 8-10 inches from surface.
Hold for 5 seconds. Repeat 10 times. Do 1 session per day.

Prone Hip Exercise

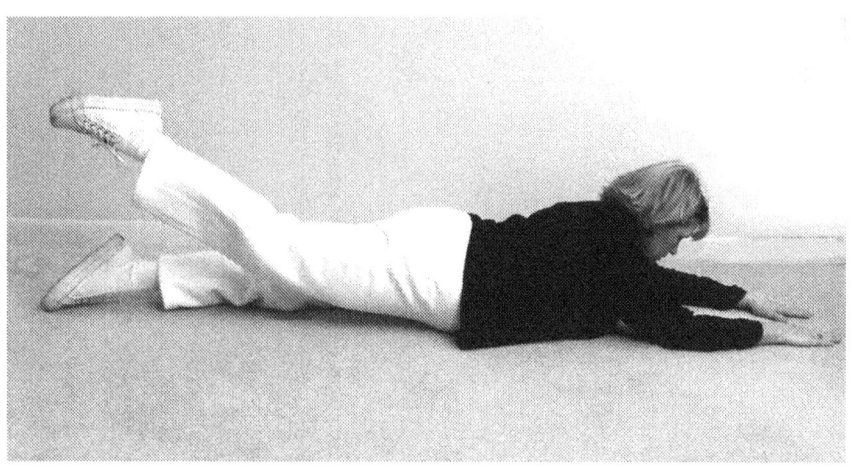

Lying on stomach, tighten muscles on front of thigh, then lift
leg 8-10 inches from surface.
Hold for 5 seconds. Repeat 10 times. Do 1 session per day.

Chapter 11

During February 1994, I tripped in the parking lot of our local grocery store and landed on the right knee. As a precaution I was sent to the emergency room for x-rays

And as always it had to be by ambulance in full c-spine on a back-board. I was pretty sure I was all right, but couldn't take the risk. Thankfully, the x-rays revealed no fracture.

At the end of May that same year my mother died. Then in October, my husband and I separated ending with a divorce that was final in 1996. We were married twenty years. The reasons for the divorce shall remain personal, but my osteoporosis was not an issue at all. (In fact, he always used to say my bones were his bones).

In May 1995, prior to the divorce being final, I found a part time job, which had not been easy. I had never worked before in my entire life. It was also against my doctor's wishes. Being a full-time wife and mother was the only role I knew. I had not even held a baby until my first daughter was born. When applying for a job I had to inform a perspective employer about my osteoporosis and restrictions. That did not go well with many places, but I eventually found a place that would hire me for my first job. In August 1995, I went back to the Mayo Clinic. I repeated all the same tests that had been done with each visit since my very first one. Blood, urine, chest x-rays, and of the bone mineral density test.

My tests once again showed deterioration to the bones with results of:

- T SPINE (Thoracic Spine)

  The bone mineral density for the left femoral neck was 0.617g/cm². This bone mineral density was 73% of the normal for my normal adjusted age and sex. And, as before, more than two standard deviations below normal adjusted for age and sex.

- L SPINE (Lumbar Spine)

  My bone density for the lumbar spine was (L 1-3) was 0.667g/cm². This was 66% of the normal adjusted for age and sex. And again, this was below the fracture threshold of 0.830g/cm². As before it was more than two standard deviations below normal adjusted for age and sex.

I informed my doctor that I continued to fall periodically and told him about the broken leg and wrist back in 1993. Fortunately, the fractures I had experienced lately seemed to be with the ribs only, but each time I fell I was transported to the hospital as a precaution.

He said there was really no change in instructions. Walking and swimming were still required and I was not allowed to lift anything over eight pounds (it had been ten). With any rib fractures, x-rays were not necessary anymore because of the frequency and exposure to radiation. Even though the radiation exposure was not that high, it was the frequency that was of concern. Every precaution to prevent other complications was important at this stage of my health.

I was to continue taking the daily calcium and vitamin D supplements. It was important to stay in contact with my primary care doctor. If any significant changes occurred, I was to call for an appointment. Otherwise my family internist could handle anything that came up. As new medications became available my local doctor would be informed.

I also let the doctor know that for the past two years I had experienced a bloated stomach, intestinal cramping and diarrhea on a regular basis. As time went by it had become worse and more often. I easily had diarrhea as much as ten to twelve times a day. There were days I couldn't even leave the house as it controlled my life. I felt like my life and health were totally out of control between this, the migraine headaches, and broken bones. While at the Mayo Clinic I mentioned this to the doctor. He suspected I suffered from Irritable Bowel Syndrome, so he had ordered some additional tests that could be done near my hometown. Only after I was diagnosed with IBS did I understand the role it played in my treatment of osteoporosis.

Irritable Bowel Syndrome, more commonly known as IBS, affects one out of every five people. It is one of the most common disorders diagnosed by primary care doctors and gastroenterologists. IBS is also referred to as a "nervous stomach," "irritable colon," or "spastic colon." It occurs in more women than men and usually begins around the age of 20. Unfortunately, there is no cure for it, but it can be controlled through diet. Following an IBS diet means learning what can prevent or trigger a spastic colon.

The doctor also told me that patients who had suffered severe endometriosis were more susceptible to irritable bowel. That didn't mean if a woman had had endometriosis she would have irritable bowel; just that a good percentage of women suffering from IBS had also suffered from endometriosis. Lucky me again! The odds were and still are, always against me. Anywhere from 30-60% of the people suffering from IBS have a low bone density. Certain drugs used to control IBS can interfere with the development and maintenance of healthy bone. Over time bone loss increases.

Abdominal pain or discomfort in association with bowel dysfunction is the main symptom. That pain is usually relieved with a bowel movement. Symptoms vary depending on the individual. Some people experience constipation (hard, difficult-to-pass, or infrequent bowel movements), others have diarrhea (frequent bowel movement), and others experience alternating between constipation and diarrhea. Many people have bloating, which is a gas build up in the intestines that may cause pain and a feeling of pressure in the abdomen. For some there may be mucous in the stool or a feeling that you have not finished a bowel movement.

Emotional stress does not cause IBS, but stress can trigger symptoms. The colon responds to stress also. Like the heart and lungs, the colon is partly controlled by the autonomic nervous system, which has been proven to respond to stress. It's not known what causes an individual to have IBS. Research suggests that people who suffer from IBS seem to have a colon that is more sensitive and reactive than usual to a variety of things, certain foods, emotions, exercise, hormones, and stress.

Irritable bowel does not cause permanent harm or damage to the intestines or lead to a serious disease such as cancer. But it can be very painful and disabling; affecting a person's ability to work, socialize, or even travel.

It's not a disease, but a functional disorder of the bowel. This means the bowel does not work like it should. The nerves and muscles are extra sensitive. For example, when you eat, the muscles may contract. These contractions can cause cramping. The nerves can be overly sensitive to the stretching of the bowel (possibly because of gas) resulting in cramping or pain as well.

IBS affects mainly the bowel (also known as the small intestine) and interferes with the function of the large intestine (the colon). The bowel is the part of the digestive system that makes and stores the stool. Syndrome means a group of symptoms occurring together characterizing a disease. IBS is a syndrome because it can cause several symptoms such as bloating, constipation, cramping, diarrhea, and gas. It also affects the movement of the stool, gas through the colon, and how fluid is absorbed. When stool remains in the colon for a long time, too much water is absorbed from it, and then it becomes hard and difficult to pass. This causes constipation. Spasms can also push the stool through the colon too fast for the fluid to be absorbed, resulting in diarrhea. Gas may also get trapped in one area or stool may collect in one place temporarily unable to move forward. If someone experiences symptoms similar to those of irritable bowel, it does not mean they have IBS. But, as a precaution they should consult their doctor.

To determine if you have Irritable Bowel Syndrome, your doctor may schedule some medical tests. A physical exam, blood tests, stool tests, an x-ray of the bowel (known as a barium enema) an endoscopy, a flexible sigmoidoscopy, or a colonoscopy are some of the tests that are used. This is usually done not to confirm IBS, but to be sure you do not have an illness or disease that causes the same symptoms as IBS.

I made an appointment with a gastroenterologist in Flagstaff, Arizona. After discussing my symptoms he felt certain I suffered from Irritable Bowel Syndrome. As a precaution, however, he scheduled me for two separate tests: an upper endoscopy and a flexible sigmoidoscopy. These tests would not confirm IBS but eliminate the possibility of a serious disease or cancer. Both procedures involved the insertion of tubes and I was not looking forward to that.

An upper endoscopy also called EGD stands for esophagogastroduodenoscopy. With the use of an endoscope, a flexible, lighted tube, would allow the doctor to look inside the esophagus, stomach, and the small part of the intestine known as the duodenum. The endoscope transmits an image on to a screen of the inside of the esophagus, stomach, and duodenum. This allows the doctor to carefully examine the lining of these organs. The scope also blows air into the stomach, expanding the folds, making it easier to examine the stomach. The doctor can see abnormalities such as inflammation or bleeding through an endoscope that would not show up well in an x-ray. Instruments can also be inserted through the scope to treat bleeding abnormalities or remove samples of tissue for further tests (biopsies).

The procedure takes approximately 20-30 minutes, but there is a one to two hour recovery because of sedation. Most people only experience a mild sore throat for a day or two after the procedure.

In my case, I was instructed not to eat or drink anything after midnight the night before my EGD procedure. Because I was to be sedated I needed to bring someone to drive me home after I was done.

When I arrived I was given a hospital gown to change in to. The doctor explained in great detail what he would be doing. An intravenous (IV) line would be placed in my right arm for a sedative that would put me in "twilight." When "twilight" was explained to me I was told that it would not put me to sleep but would block the memory in my brain, leaving me with no recollection of the procedure once it was over. I told him to give me a lot of the "twilight" medicine because I didn't want to know it at the moment even if I would not remember it later. Before giving me the sedative, a device with a hole in the center of it was placed in my mouth. The hole was to pass a thin, flexible, lighted tube called an endoscope through. The device was to prevent my jaws from locking or my mouth from clamping shut. Next to me was a monitor that would show images on the screen from the endoscope put down my throat. If the doctor saw any abnormalities he would insert an instrument into the scope and remove tissue samples for further testing. He would also blow air into my stomach, making it easier to examine.

Once the EGD procedure was over I stayed in recovery for approximately an hour and a half before being released to go home. Tissue samples had been taken so I had some tenderness deep inside my chest. I ended up with a sore throat for several days.

Two weeks after having an upper endoscopy I returned to Flagstaff for a flexible sigmoidoscopy. It was definitely something I had not looked forward to. Without the aid of a sedative, a scope was inserted up my rectum to the last part of my colon.

A "flexible sigmoidoscopy" is a procedure where a flexible, lighted tube is inserted into the rectum and slowly guided up into the colon. The scope transmits an image on to a monitor that allows the doctor to look at the inside of the large intestine from the rectum through the last part of the colon. That last part of the colon is commonly called the sigmoid or descending colon. The scope also blows air into these organs, which inflates them making it easier for the doctor to examine.

Doctors often use this procedure to find the cause of abdominal pain, constipation, or diarrhea. It also allows them to look for early signs of cancer in the descending colon and rectum. By doing this procedure the doctor can see abnormal growths, bleeding, inflammation, and ulcers in the descending colon and rectum. If anything unusual is observed in the rectum or last part of the colon, the doctor can insert an instrument through the scope and remove a piece of tissue for testing (biopsy).

Because air is blown in, the patient may feel some discomfort in the lower abdomen, experiencing a feeling of pressure or cramping. The patient will feel better once the air leaves the colon. A flexible sigmoidoscopy takes approximately twenty minutes. Because no sedative is given, the patient is able to drive home.

I was told to have clear liquids only beginning 24 hours before the test. I was not to have anything after midnight the night before the actual procedure. I also had to drink a quart of liquid, which reminded me of straight lemon juice without water or sugar. It was very acidic, tasted awful, and was difficult swallow. Its purpose was that it was a very strong laxative.

Once again, upon my arrival, I was told to change into a hospital gown. The doctor came in and explained that he would insert a flexible, lighted tube up my rectum and into the lower portion of my colon. Just like before, there was a monitor to help him see inside. If he saw anything unusual, tissue samples would be taken for testing.

I had to lie on my left side while this test was being done. I remember once the air was blown in, it was extremely uncomfortable. A nurse was holding my hand and I was squeezing very hard. She told me my squeeze was hurting her and I remember commenting she had workman's comp. That death grip was the only thing helping me get through it. Once the doctor was finished looking inside I remember the air being sucked out and a feeling of relief.

Once the procedure was over, I was allowed to go home. The doctor told me he had taken some samples of polyps for testing as a precautionary measure but thought they would come out fine. I would also have quite a bit of gas for the rest of the day and should refrain from carbonated drinks and foods that create gas.

About ten days later I learned both procedures had come out just fine. The biopsies showed no cancer or other disease. I clearly had irritable bowel syndrome. I was told there is no cure for IBS but it can be controlled to a certain point with diet.

If three large meals a day cause discomfort, then try six smaller meals. Large amounts of wheat, rye, barley, chocolate, milk products, alcohol, carbonated drinks, and beverages with caffeine have also been associated with a worsening of IBS symptoms. It may help if meals are low in fat and high in carbohydrates (pasta, rice, whole-grain breads, and cereals), fruits and vegetables. Dairy products may cause IBS symptoms to flare up. Yogurt is tolerated more than any other dairy product because it contains bacteria that supply the enzyme needed to digest lactose (the sugar found in milk products).

When that doctor told me all this, suddenly my past came back to me. When I was eleven years old I was told to refrain from dairy products because I couldn't tolerate them, but there was no diagnosis named "IBS." A lack of calcium intake had been a contributing factor in my acquiring osteoporosis.

That also explained the problem with some of the medications I had been trying for the osteoporosis. Because of the constant diarrhea, the medicine went right through me including the calcium and vitamin D. My body never had a chance to absorb any of it. The doctor also gave me a prescription to take one half hour before a meal. It was to calm the colon down and help prevent the muscles from going into spasms. With time I learned what foods would trigger a reaction. Eventually I learned the early symptoms when I had too much of something, and could stop before going into an IBS routine. After a year I was able to discontinue the mediation and control my IBS with diet.

Along with changes in the diet, certain medications can help with IBS symptoms. Your primary care doctor can discuss those medications with you and select the one most suited for you and your symptoms.

Picture of the Digestive System[15]

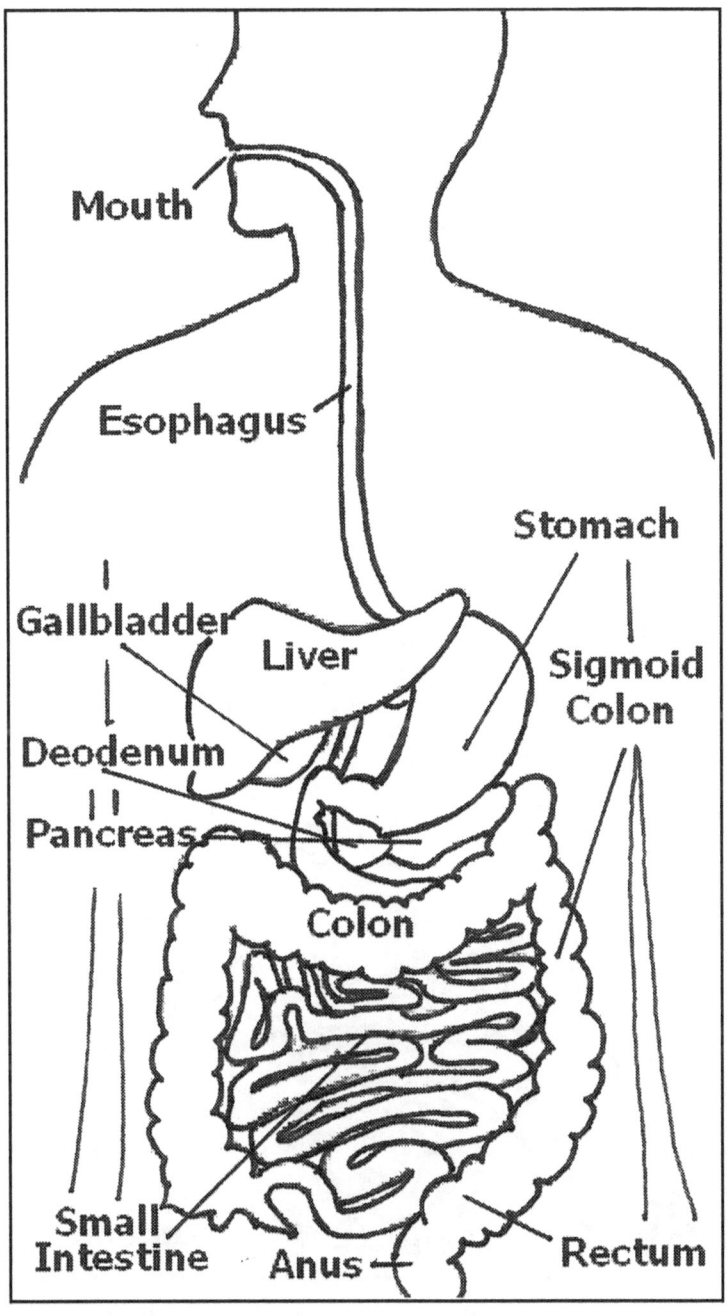

---

[15] Courtesy of National Digestive Diseases Information Clearinghouse.

Picture For Flexible Endoscopy[16]

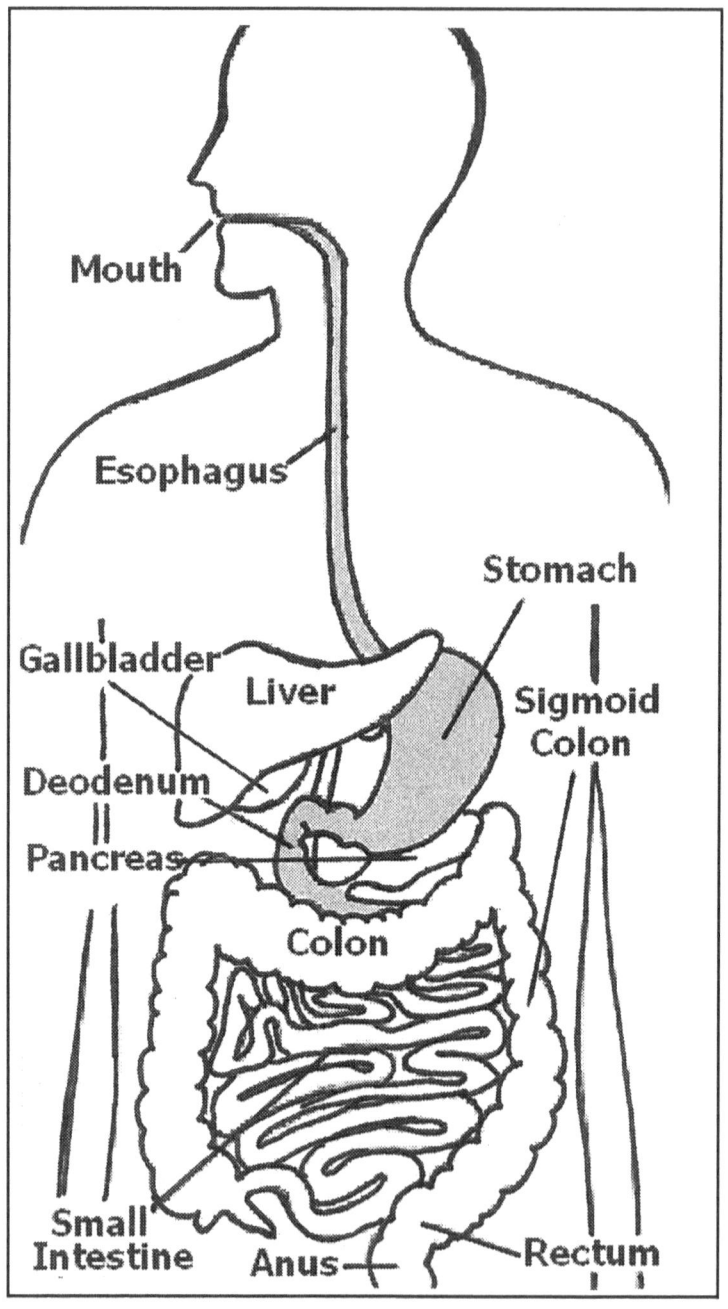

Shaded area shows the route for the Flexible Endoscopy

---

[16] Courtesy of National Digestive Diseases Information Clearinghouse.

Picture For Sigmoidoscopy[17]

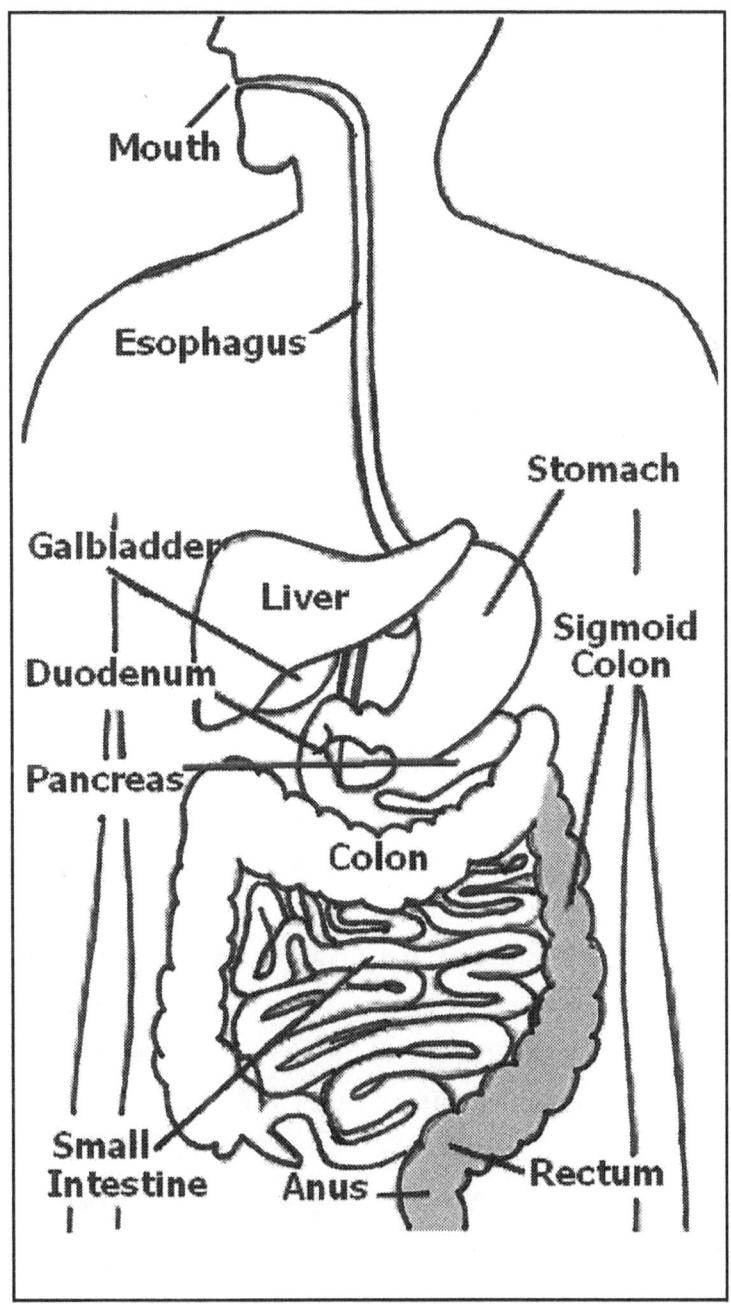

Shaded area shows the route for the Sigmoidoscopy.

[17] Courtesy of National Digestive Diseases Information Clearinghouse.

Chapter 12

I eventually had two more part-time jobs each paying better than the previous one, but the physical strength was too much for me. My primary care doctor also stated because I suffered from severe osteoporosis that I shouldn't work. I was a risk to myself physically, and a liability to an employer. The time came when I had to realize I was not able to work anymore.

In July 1996, when my divorce was final, I was granted lifetime alimony unless I died or remarried because of my health condition. However, I lost the insurance that my husband had on me through his employer, and I could not afford a Cobra plan to maintain the insurance because it cost over five hundred dollars a month. This became a very major problem financially. I was still continuing to break ribs on a regular basis, but fortunately had not broken any major bones since 1993. If I did it would have been financially devastating. I continued walking and swimming as much as I could. Throughout all this time I also continued to break ribs, fall, and have trips to the hospital. Each ambulance trip and visit to the emergency room cost money and I had no insurance. Irritable bowel seemed to reappear as well — most likely due to the financial stress as medical bills began to grow. I also had the periodic migraines that required treatment. More bills!

In September, I fell again landing on the right knee. It hurt quite a bit and there was an abrasion to the knee. Once again, there were x-rays but no fractures were seen. There was damage to the soft tissue so the knee was immobilized. Weight on it was "as tolerated." It would be a few more years down the road before I understood why I kept falling so much.

Then in 1997 I had to move. I bought a smaller house on a much smaller lot. I could not take my Doughboy swimming pool because the new backyard was not large enough in width, so swimming ended completely. I couldn't afford a new pool in ground or above ground. The local community pool was only open three months out of the year if it didn't have problems.

I had joined the Yavapai County Sheriff's Office Search and Rescue. Their purpose was to find lost, injured, or deceased individuals using various resources. There were trackers (hikers), 4x4 (four wheel drive), mounted (horseback riders), swift-water rescues, and mountain climbers. All members had to pass a background check and be state certified. On my application I put down my severe osteoporosis and that I was unable to participate in any of these units, but could work in base camp doing paper work. After becoming state certified I was assigned to the command post working with deputies and others regarding radio communications and logistics.

Even though I had very good friends to do things with, I had been so frustrated not being able to work and be out and about more. At least this gave me an outlet to do something worthwhile that helped others and allowed me to socialize with different people.

Early in 1998, a friend had her elderly father living in fully contained guest quarters off their main house. He had a caregiver who came in each weekday morning to prepare his breakfast, make the bed, and do minor household chores. The caregiver went on vacation and never came back to work. Knowing my income had been drastically reduced by the divorce, my friend asked if I would like to care for her father. So, I once again became employed. It was only for three hours a day, Monday through Friday, but it gave me extra income and helped to ease the pinch. It also required no lifting or strenuous work so my osteoporosis was not compromised. It gave me a chance to earn some extra money and be doing something constructive. I felt like part of the human race again.

That May, when my youngest daughter turned eighteen, graduated from high school and moved out, my lifestyle changed again. Suddenly with no one around I was lifting more than I should. I began doing more physical things than the doctor would have approved of. There was a lot of physical back pain because of the strain put on it. Rib fractures began to increase. I was living alone with things that just had to be done. A limited budget prevented me from hiring outside help. I could no longer keep my annual visits at the Mayo Clinic. I also worried about getting help if I fell. There had always been someone at home if that happened in the past. I needed to be more careful than ever.

In 1999, I met my future husband, Randy, who was also in Search and Rescue and seventeen years older than me. I didn't know then that we would end up married. I had met him at the meetings, but never gave it another thought. Going down that road never crossed my mind, but he swept me off my feet and there was no going back. He was a volunteer Intermediate Emergency Medical Technician (IEMT) with the Sedona Fire Department and having had both his hips replaced a few years back, he was very compassionate about my medical conditions. Randy moved in to my house in May of 2000.

Around 5:30 in the afternoon on November 4, 2000, I had just come out of a movie theater in Sedona, Arizona, with my friend B.J. There was evidence it had rained during the movie but was not raining at the time we exited. Just as B.J. said to be careful my foot became caught in an uneven crack in the sidewalk and I fell. Of all places, I had fallen in the handicapped area. I told B.J. I was hurt and needed someone to call 911. B.J. went and asked the theater to call 911 and relayed to them what had just happened.

Ironically, the movie we had just seen had been about giving back and helping others. Many of the people who exited with us were more than willing to offer any kind of assistance. A woman I had never met took off her beautiful leather jacket, rolled it up in a ball and placed it under my head to keep my head dry since the ground was wet and had puddles. Another person, a complete stranger, knelt down and just held my hand. Someone else offered to call a family member, which B.J. had already done. There was such an outpouring of truly wanting to help and genuine concern.

Once the ambulance arrived, the medics cut my jeans so they could get a better look at the injury. I was then put into a full c-spine precaution (again!) and transported to an emergency room facility in Sedona. The paramedics who had treated me were from the same fire station Randy worked out of.

I don't know how fast Randy drove, but he was waiting for me when we arrived at the emergency room. I was just thankful he was there.

Before the x-rays were taken I was given pain medication just like every other time in the past. Then x-rays were taken of my right knee, neck, lower back, and right shoulder. The x-rays revealed a displaced fractured right patella (kneecap). I was informed that the emergency room doctor had spoken to my orthopedic doctor. I would soon be transferred to Cottonwood by ambulance for surgery. The emergency room doctor had also been requested to do preoperative lab work. Before being reloaded in to the ambulance for transport I was given a large dose of Versed. A few minutes later after the Versed had kicked in the emergency room doctor straightened out my leg. I never felt a thing. That medication had put me in "la-la land." I was then transported from to Sedona to Cottonwood but barely remember the trip. Since x-rays had been done I did not need a c-spine for the transport to Cottonwood and I was very grateful.

After a 25-minute drive we arrived at the hospital and I was admitted to the floor with a private room. Nurses kept coming in and out gathering medical information etc. Registration came in to confirm all my personal financial history, current family history, mailing address, etc. The doctor arrived and explained the surgical procedure, which required titanium screws being placed in the knee to hold it together. As with any surgery, complications were also mentioned such as bleeding, infections, temporary or permanent nerve damage, muscular atrophy, a permanent loss of some mobility, and post-traumatic arthritis. There was the fear of hardware failure along with not gaining full strength in the knee. The healing process would take at least eight to ten weeks because of the osteoporosis and physical therapy was required to gain the most mobility possible.

Because of the threat of blood clots, a blood thinner, Coumadin was required. Next was the anesthesiologist who explained his role during my surgery. Finally around 10:30 that evening I was wheeled down to surgery.

I returned to my room around midnight with a morphine IV drip. The next morning when I was more aware I realized there were two drains coming out of my knee. The incision had been closed with staples and when I saw them I thought I would faint. When did they start doing that? I had on surgical hose and was in horrendous pain. I prayed that this would never happen again.

Later that morning the doctor came in to tell me how the surgery had gone. He said that the fracture had been in the middle of the patella with a fragment of bone measuring two centimeters wide and two centimeters in vertical length. There were also fragments in the surrounding area and a tear in the capsule. Three titanium screws were inserted and all had excellent fixation. Two drains were placed deep within the knee through separate incisions.

Two days after the surgery had been performed the doctor removed the drains. First, he told me to find a focal point on the wall, take a deep breath a not to lose that focal point. At that point he pulled out the drains. Oh My God! It was painful and felt like something had been ripped out of me (which is exactly what had happened). Seven years later I still have the scars from where the drains had been.

The following day I was finally released. Back in the comfort of my home I was taking medication for the pain and using a walker to get around. The right leg had to be elevated above my heart as much as possible. The knee immobilizer could be adjusted but not removed. I also had to have weekly blood tests to check my clotting time since I was on Coumadin to prevent any blood clots. As time went by the doctor gradually changed the pain medication and dosage as the healing process continued.

Just after Thanksgiving we had to go to a wedding in Florence, Arizona. You don't realize the difficulty handicapped people have in traveling until you become one of them. In my case, it was temporary — at least I hoped it was. Everything was a struggle, from taking a shower, dressing up (since I wore loose clothing at home to accommodate the immobilizer), to getting in and out of a vehicle.

Next, I had to face Christmas, which was usually my favorite time of year. My dear friend B.J. took me to Scottsdale so we could do our annual Christmas shopping. By then I was using crutches. I had made a list of items or had specific ideas. But I swear it didn't matter what we wanted, it was always at the opposite end of the mall. I didn't even want to know how many times we walked that mall back and forth. I thought I would die from pain and exhaustion and almost prayed I would. By the time I was back home and in bed, my knee was swollen and it took a couple of days to recover. If B. J. and I had been thinking, we should have divided it up in to a couple of trips rather than one very long day. I also should have been in a wheelchair.

Physical therapy is a very important part of recovery and is often overlooked by the patient. Physical therapists are experts in movement and function and help people of all ages, from infants to the elderly depending on the need. With the help of a physical therapist, they will set up a specialized program just for you. The purpose of your individualized work out program is to help restore lost mobility and strength, increase your fitness, and reduce pain. They will teach you the necessary exercises and how to use your body properly to increase recovery and to decrease the chances of further injury due to conditions resulting from diseases or injuries. Anyone who has suffered an injury affecting bones, ligaments, or muscles can truly benefit from specialized physical therapy.

Physical therapy can mean the difference in how much mobility the patient is able to get back after a traumatic injury. As important as it is to work with a physical therapist, it is just as important to follow up with exercises the patient is requested to do at home. This can make a big difference in how quickly one recovers.

Physical therapy started very quickly at the local hospital and was extremely painful and grueling. I had electrical stimulation prior to each workout. Exercises consisted of stairs, using a treadmill, a ball and lying on my back and walking down a wall, forcing the right knee to bend as much as possible. I had to lie on my back, place my foot flat against the wall and slide it down. The goal was to eventually be able to have a bend that measured 135 degrees but I only got to one hundred and ten degrees. There were all kinds of leg lifts with ankle weights that really tested my endurance. I also had to put a towel under my foot and pull it up, bending the knee as much as possible.

Some of the exercises might have sounded weak to someone else (especially to an athlete), but I wasn't a physically active person and the leg had lost a lot of muscle strength during recovery due to lack of mobility. Every person is different in his or her injury and recovery process. I did try to always exceed the required number of repetitions when doing my exercises. I wanted to get back to my "normal" way of living as quickly as possible. After each therapy session an ice pack was placed on the area for 20 minutes to keep down the inflammation. Pain was tolerable since I took a prescription half an hour before going to therapy. That was on the advice of my doctor or I never would have survived the workouts. The therapy sessions at the hospital were three times a week for one and a half hours. On the other days I did the weight lifts and the wall walk at home followed by ice for 20 minutes. Finally, after five and a half months of therapy the doctor released me.

Full Cervical Spinal Stabilization Again.

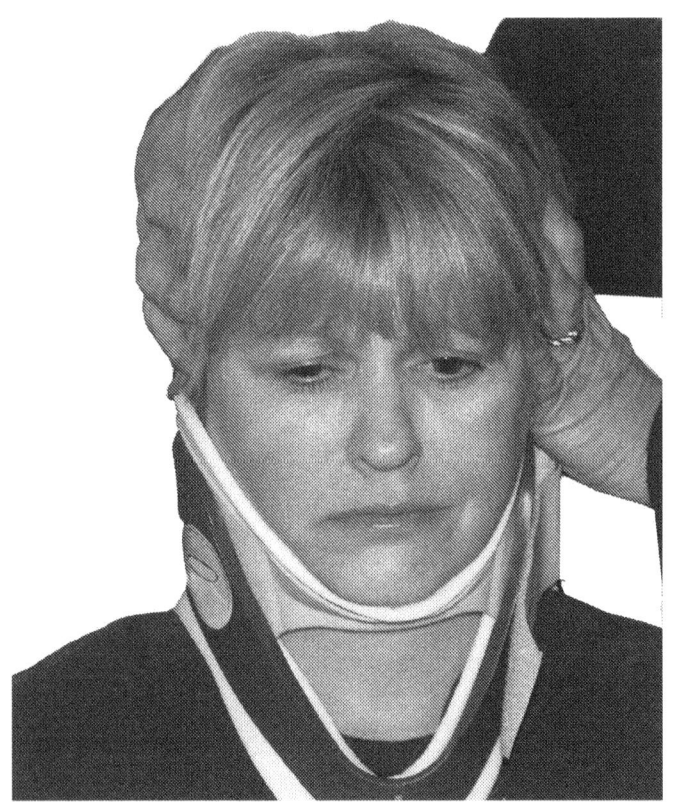

Once again, secured on a backboard for transport to the hospital.

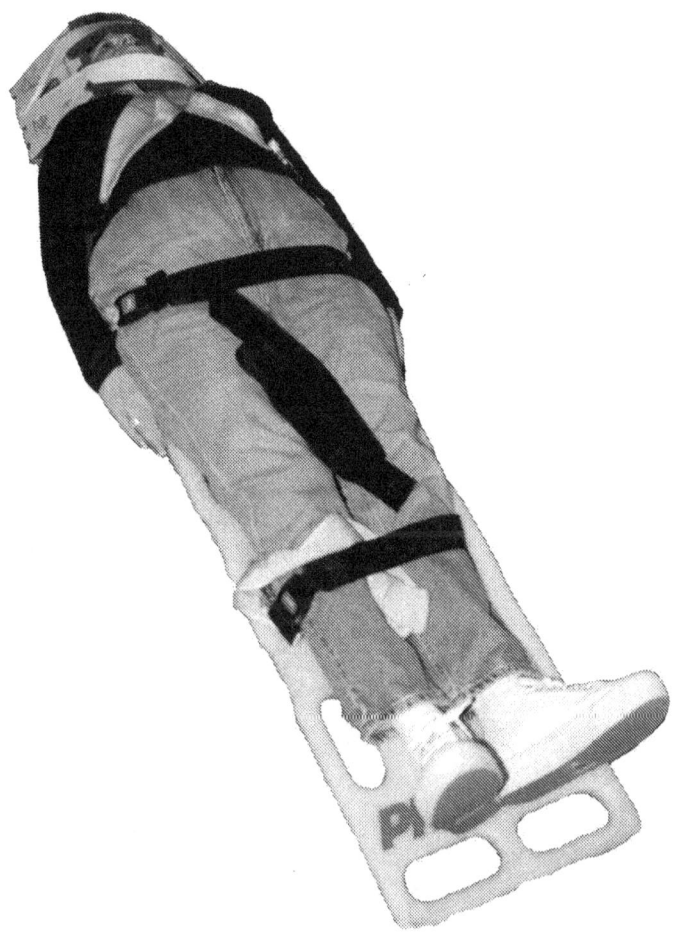

Normal Right Patella (Kneecap)

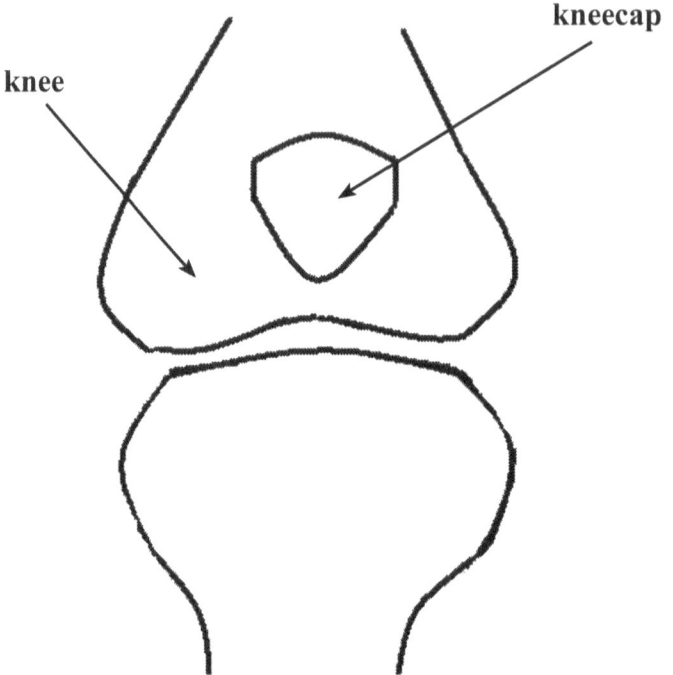

kneecap

knee

Fractured Right Patella (Kneecap)

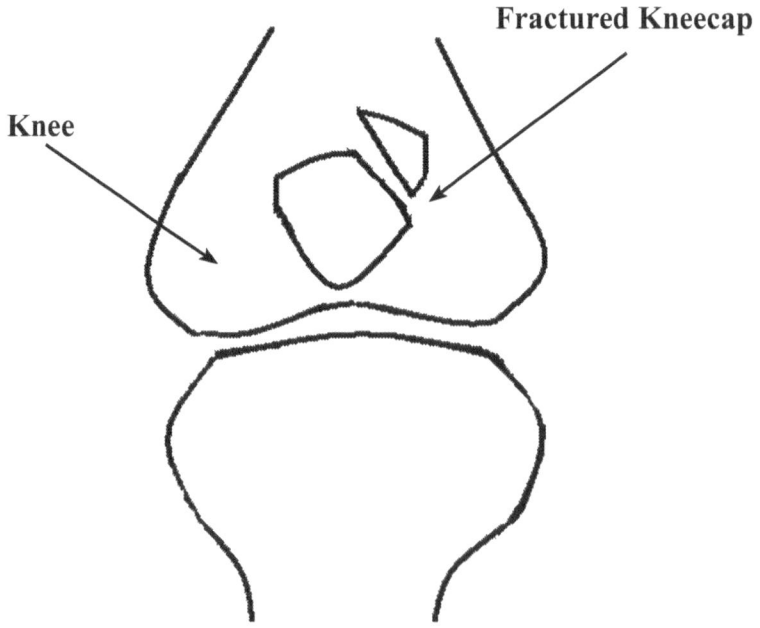

Fractured Kneecap

Knee

Knee Immobilizer

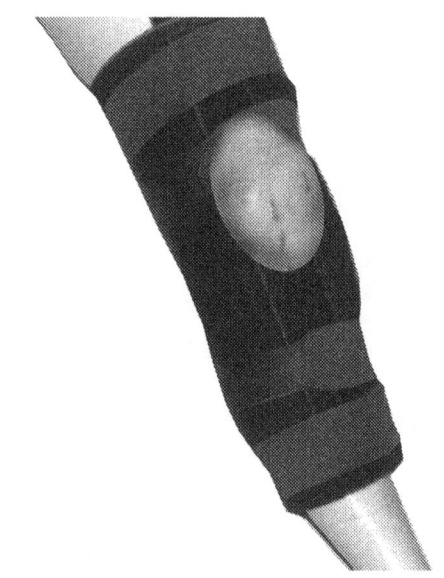

Mobility Assistance

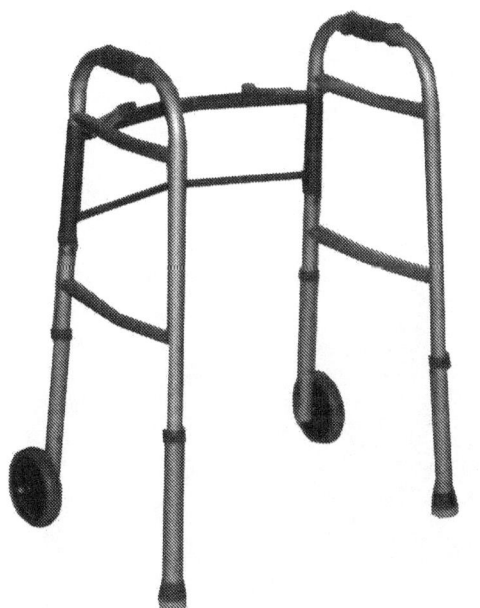

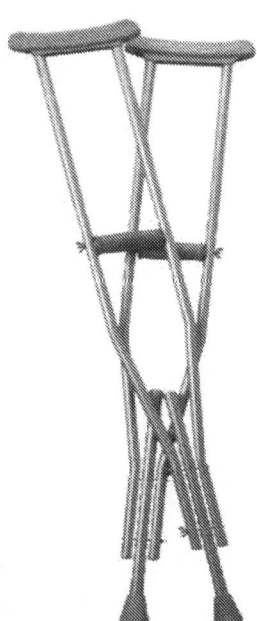

Walker   **Crutches**

Physical Therapy Exercises For The Right Patella.

<u>Stretching</u>

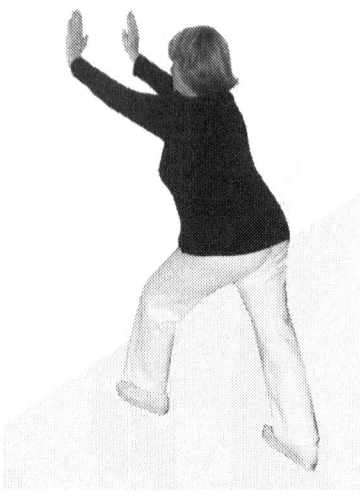

**Keep back leg straight, with heel on floor and turned slightly outward.
Lean in to wall till stretch is felt.
Hold <u>60</u> seconds. Repeat <u>5</u> times. Do <u>1</u> session per day.**

<u>Knee Wall Slides</u>

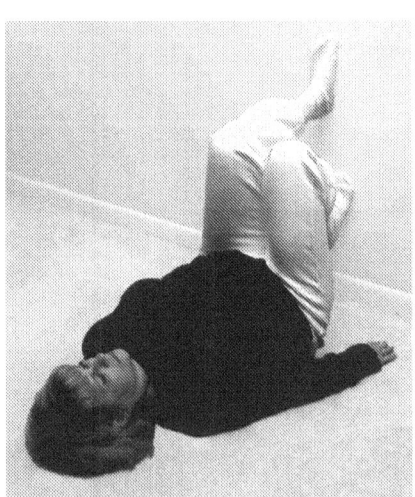

**Slowly walk or slide foot on wall towards the floor
until a stretch is felt in the knee.
Hold for <u>60</u> seconds. Repeat <u>10</u> times. Do <u>2</u> sessions per day.**

Straight Leg Raise

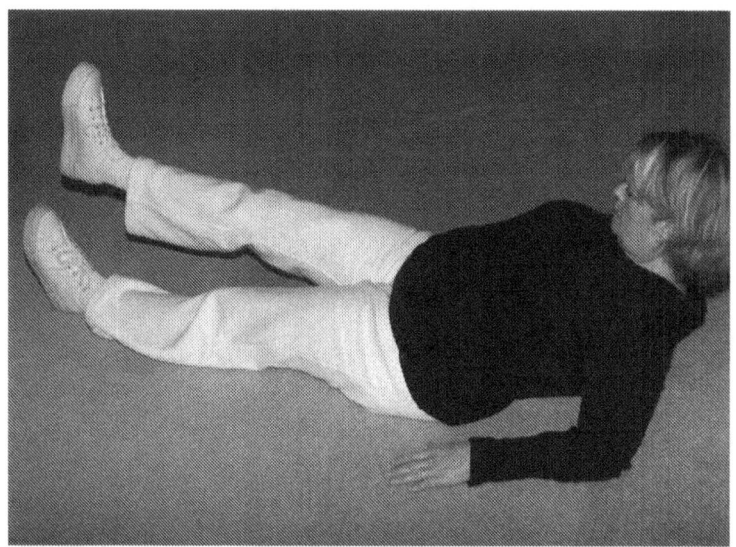

Rest on forearms; tighten muscles on front of thigh.
Then lift leg 8-10 inches from surface, keeping knee locked.
Hold for 5 seconds. Repeat 10 times. Do 1 session per day.

Strengthening

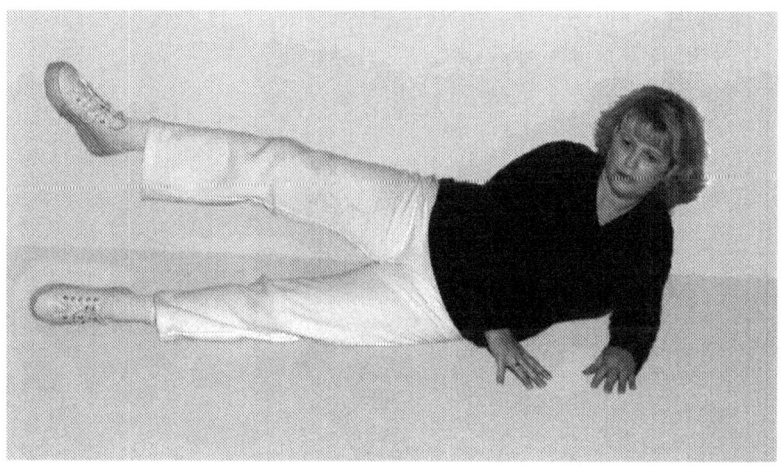

Lying on your side, tighten muscles on your front thigh.
Lift leg 8-10 inches from surface.
Hold for 5 seconds. Repeat 10 times. Do 1 session per day.

Prone Hip Extension

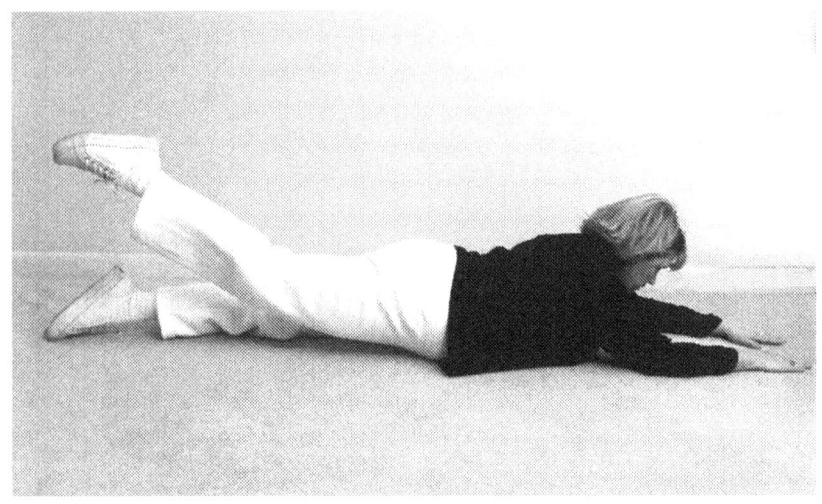

Lying on stomach, tighten muscles on front of thigh,
then lift leg 8-10 from surface, keeping knee locked.
Hold 5 seconds. Repeat 10 times. Do 1 session per day.

Side-Lying Hip Extension

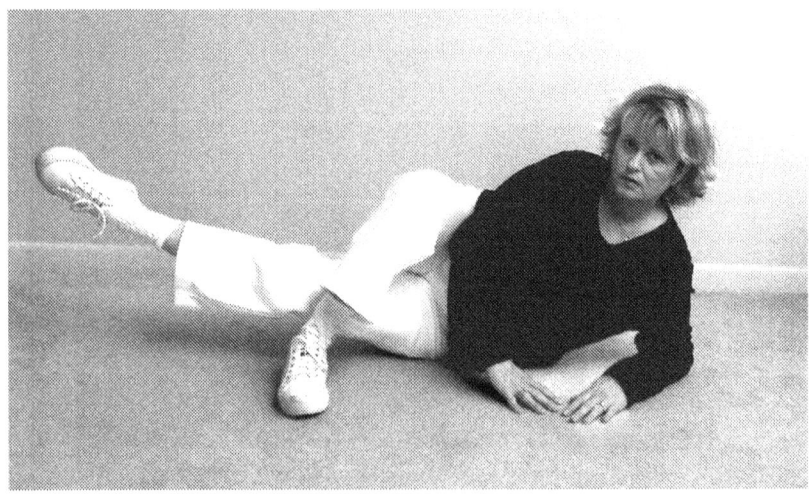

Lying on side, tighten muscles on front thigh.
Then lift leg 8-10 inches from surface.
Hold 5 seconds. Repeat 10 times. Do 1 session per day.

Chapter 13

In June of 2001, I became employed at the Camp Verde Marshal's Office in Camp Verde, Arizona. It was only by some miracle that I was awarded the position as Record's Clerk. I had seen an advertisement in the local paper for the job description and thought I might be able to handle a desk job. It would be a regular income including insurance. Randy and I were to be married in September and my lifetime alimony would end at that time due to a remarriage.

After extensive testing, interviews, psychological examinations, and a polygraph, I began work on July 16, 2001. As the records clerk, I entered citations and arrests into the computer, and prepared felony files for Grand Jury indictments along with numerous other duties.

The Marshal's Office was aware of my medical condition and was more than willing to accommodate my limitations. I could not climb ladders in the records vault or lift heavy boxes that held case files.

As a town employee I would receive medical, dental, and vision insurance; something I had been without for five years. I was also able to acquire supplemental insurance. Believe me, I took that opportunity and ran with it. I knew this might be my one and only chance to get this additional insurance and if I left my employment I could maintain any policies I had purchased. The payments would be deducted out of my checking account rather than from my payroll check. Also at the time of purchase, the premium was based on the age of the policyholder and would never increase as long as the policy was owned without interruption.

By planning for the present and the future I purchased accident, cancer, disability, intensive care, and personal recovery policies. Several years later I purchased life insurance for Randy and myself. These policies — if they were ever redeemed — would help towards any deductibles that had not been met.

I still continued to fall, even at work. Most of the falls resulted in fractured ribs, but I kept my mouth shut for fear of losing my job. When I did fall in front of someone I made light of it saying I was just fine, knowing I needed this job and the insurance desperately. There were a few times that I fell in front of the Animal Control Officer but I begged her to keep quiet. I was afraid I would be considered a risk and I loved my job and what I did.

Then on Sunday, May 25, 2003, I experienced the worst fracture yet. It was the Memorial Day weekend. We owned a large fifth wheel recreational vehicle at the time and had gone camping for the long weekend near Happy Jack, Arizona, located a little over an hour away from home. Happy Jack was a roadside town between Strawberry and Payson in the high country. We camped about five miles from Happy Jack back in the woods. Randy was in the bathroom showering and I was standing on the stairs between the bedroom and living room. Our black Labrador was on the stairs with me. As I turned to go upstairs, he thought I was going to go downstairs and went right between my legs causing me to fall down four stairs. I knew immediately that my leg was broken. My back and neck were also in pain but I kept that to myself. I knew that would require a helicopter instead of an ambulance, and I wasn't doing that. When Randy finally came out he asked what I was doing on the floor and I told him, the dog tripped me, I was hurt, and the right leg was badly broken.

After assessing me, I had him drag me to the couch so I could get off the floor and away from the dog. I also had him help me change out of my pajama bottoms and into shorts. I did not want my pajamas cut off. He also started me on oxygen before leaving me to get help. Since he is a medic he always has a medical supply pack with him whether it is in the car, truck, trailer, etc.

Once Randy was dressed he drove about five miles to Happy Jack where the Forest Service had a small office. The Forest Service Ranger followed Randy back to our campsite so that she could give accurate instructions for the ambulance. When they returned, I informed them how bad my back and neck really hurt because I was scared of permanent damage. After the Ranger spoke to me she order a helicopter for transport since that is protocol for possible neck injury, then went out to the main road to wait for the ambulance and lead them in to our campsite. Meanwhile, Randy began preparing the trailer for the trip home.

Once the paramedics and ambulance dispatched out of Strawberry arrived, they began working on me. They could not get an IV started to help the pain and they were very concerned about my breathing. Apparently they were not hearing the proper breath sounds in one lung. A helicopter had been dispatched out of Payson and took about fifteen minutes to arrive. However we were in such a remote area the helicopter had to find a landing zone about six miles away. After trying several more times to start an IV the paramedics decided the lack of breath sound was more important and stopped trying to start the IV. The ambulance then had to transport me to the landing zone. Prior to loading me on to the helicopter they tried one more time to start an IV without success. I was then loaded on to the helicopter and flown to

Flagstaff Medical Center. While in the air on the third try, the flight nurse was able to get an IV going and pumped in lots of morphine. They were also in contact with the hospital the entire time.

It was a very eerie feeling laying on a gurney so high up in the sky. I kept asking if we were clear from the trees. Around two o' clock in the afternoon we arrived on the roof of the hospital in Flagstaff. It was a very secure feeling to be on solid ground again. Despite my pain and discomfort, the flight crew could not have been nicer or gentler in their treatment.

The Emergency Room doctor came right away and ordered numerous x-rays and tests. Once the x-rays were read he said I had a tibial plateau fracture. That was a fracture of the weight bearing bone in my right leg. I was given more morphine and put in a private room. I was scheduled for surgery later that evening but ended up not having it until six o'clock the next morning. That same evening I called the Marshal's Office to tell them what happened and that I wouldn't be back to work for quite a while.

I don't remember the next couple of days following surgery. They had me on a morphine drip every six minutes along with injections every four hours. On the end of the third day I started to become more aware and asked why I had been so drugged. I was told the pain would have been so unbearable— that was the procedure to keep the patient comfortable.

The doctor told me large screws had been put in to hold the bone together. He also said that my osteoporosis was so bad that when he was drilling the screws in, one went right through and out again. Also, a piece of bone had pierced a nerve in my leg. To this day it is still numb in that area. I was told it would be a very long recovery for two reasons; first, the type of fracture, and second, the osteoporosis slows down the healing process. If I wanted to have any normal use of the leg again I would have to follow all strictly ordered instructions.

After four days I was finally released to go home and to be on bed rest for the first six weeks. I had to use a wheelchair for the bathroom, getting meals and any other mobility. Not one fraction of weight could be placed on the leg. Putting weight on the leg too early could sacrifice walking normal for the rest of my life. That was an extremely long and painful time. I learned all kinds of home decorating tips as I lay in bed watching television. I could hardly wait to be completely healed and have some fun decorating.

My husband still had to work each day I was on my own. Prior to leaving in the morning, he would set out whatever I needed for breakfast and lunch to make it easier for me. I could not even stand up to get a glass for a drink or a plate for food out of the cupboard, so all of that was left on the kitchen counter where I could grab it while in the wheelchair. I had two cats at the time and one of them, Muffin, a gray Tabby, insisted on being my nurse. I cannot even count the number of times I accidentally rode over her tail with the wheelchair when I tried to maneuver my way down the hall, into the bathroom or the kitchen. My hallway is not very wide so it was a difficult task, plus I was in an adolescent size wheelchair because I am just over five feet tall it fit. The adult size was too large for me to maneuver and did not fit going down the hall.

The cat screamed and I practically cried every time. But I never broke her tail nor did she have a crook in it as a result. She was just trying to be close to me. I finally solved the problem by putting her in my lap as we went down the hall to the kitchen. I never did learn how to drive that wheelchair properly (I swear you need a license to drive it). And once I was totally recovered there was a lot of painting done to finally make good use of all those home-decorating shows I had watched.

Having to be on bed rest for the first six weeks was not without complications. I began having a difficult time breathing and it hurt to inhale or exhale. Having barely survived a pulmonary embolism many years ago, I immediately called my doctor in Sedona. And my friend Bobby took me in. They ordered a lung scan at the lab in their facility, but had a very hard time getting the IV in me. After about literally eight tries, they said they would give it one more try, and if that failed I would have to be transported by ambulance to the hospital in Cottonwood where an anesthesiologist would have to do it. I was tired, felt horrible, and just wanted it all over with. They got the IV in, did the scan, and found out I had severe pneumonia and that I would have to be hospitalized in Flagstaff since my doctor for my fracture was up there. I began to cry and begged to be allowed to recover at home. I didn't care what I had to do and not do, I just wanted to be at home where I was more comfortable.

Pneumonia, the sixth leading cause of death in the United States is an infection caused by bacteria, fungi, or viruses and affects one or both lungs. Like osteoporosis, pneumonia does not discriminate when it comes to age, however, young children and the elderly are more at risk.

People who develop pneumonia may usually experience symptoms similar to a cold. Chest pain when breathing, chills, coughing, coughing up discolored mucous, difficulty when inhaling and exhaling a breath, headaches, high fevers, and loss of appetite are also symptoms associated with and experienced by a person with pneumonia.

The doctor may suspect pneumonia when using a stethoscope to listen to a patient's breathing; they hear coarse or crackling sounds. Sometimes a patient can even feel or hear the coarse breathing in their chest. A chest x-ray will confirm if an individual has pneumonia. If a person is hospitalized for other reasons, then a clear diagnosis may be difficult to obtain. A lung scan may be requested to eliminate the possibility of a pulmonary embolism.

That was exactly what happened to me. I had surgery and when I finally came home I was not able to be mobile. Because I was down in bed fluid began to build up in my lungs and I experienced some of the symptoms just mentioned above. Some of those symptoms were similar to a pulmonary embolism like the chest pains and difficulty in breathing. Knowing my history of pulmonary embolism, the doctor was not going to take any risks. So the lung scan was done and fortunately I had pneumonia, the lesser of two evils.

After phone conferences, strict orders and medications were prescribed, I was finally allowed to go home. Every three days, however, I had to go in for x-rays to monitor the healing process of the pneumonia. If there was no change or things worsened I would be admitted into the hospital— period— no discussion. You can bet I followed those rules. I coughed when I was supposed to, I moved around more than I should have and I breathed in to a machine to build up the strength in my lungs. If the doctor said to do ten, I did twenty. There was no way I was going back into the hospital. Eventually, after about three weeks I was considered fully recovered from the pneumonia.

As far back as I can remember I have had a complex about cleanliness. Because of this I vacuumed, scrubbed bathrooms, and mopped daily, even while working. I was so proud when I learned how to do it in a wheelchair shortly after recovering from the pneumonia. This also relieved Randy from another household chore since everything was his responsibility after coming home from work.

It became quite depressing to stay in the house continuously. I could not go in the family room because you had to step down. The laundry room and pantry were off of that room, so they were also off limits. I couldn't go outside in the backyard because of the family room step as well as stepping down on to the patio. Also the backyard was and still is not handicap friendly. In fact, every door exiting our house has at least a three-inch drop.

Once Randy would get home he would maneuver my wheelchair and we would sit out on the patio under our gazebo and have a happy hour. This allowed me to get some fresh air. There were also times he would lift me up in to his truck, put the wheelchair in the back and take off for Phoenix or Prescott. That was only after the initial six weeks were up. It felt great to get out of the house. I truly understood how some older people never recover from a serious illness or injury, but die instead. The depression really gets a hold of you.

Physical therapy began the end of June only not at the hospital. Ironically, it was a physical therapy office owned by the therapist who had discovered my osteoporosis all those years ago in Sedona and had told me to have my doctor send me to the Mayo Clinic. Since I was unable to drive, my husband had to get me there and back and also assist in getting me in and out of his vehicle. The therapist was supposed to work on my range of motion. But physical therapy did not last long because of piercing pain on the side of my leg. After numerous visits and x-rays with the doctor it was determined that a screw was piercing a nerve. Because of the severe osteoporosis, the bone was so porous it had caused the screw to slip. And I would have to wait till it had been twelve weeks since the original surgery before the doctor could go back in and remove the screws. This was to guarantee that the bones had healed, especially since osteoporosis slows down the healing process. All this time the pain was awful and I was still on regular doses of pain medication.

After eight weeks I was able to use the walker and I started to do more around the house. I had a pocket on it and could work my way to the laundry room and pantry. I was able to put food items stored in the pantry in to the pocket and began cooking again. Cooking is something I love and it relaxes me. It felt good to surprise Randy with dinner that first night. And I was able to start doing laundry again. I could not carry a laundry basket because I needed both hands on the walker (I still could not put weight on the right leg but hopped on my left), but I could carry a plastic grocery bag on my wrist with clothes to wash and dry.

Most people have no idea how good it feels to be doing normal household chores after not being able to do them for a long time, even if the approach is different than normal. I began to feel useful again because there were times when I wondered if it would ever happen. Those days of doing chores left me totally exhausted from doing really very little, but I loved it. I had accomplished something constructive.

Now that I was using a walker I was allowed to drive if I drove with the left foot. That was quite interesting. I had to remember to brake with left foot. In an emergency I could not slam it down with the right. The ability to drive gave me another sense of freedom. I drove to the local grocery store, used my cell phone to call them inside and asked for an electric cart to be brought to my vehicle. I had a handicap tag so I was parked in handicap. I was starting to really get out in the world again. That first time in the grocery store I felt like a kid in a candy shop. Once the cart's basket was full and I had checked out, an employee went out to my van with me, loaded the groceries, and took the cart back. I had all refrigerator and freezer items placed together. When I got home, after numerous trips of filling the walker pouch I had the perishable groceries in the house. The rest sat in the van until Randy came home and unloaded it for me. I also learned to do more frequent shopping trips buying fewer items to make it easier, but the first trip was a mega-shopping spree.

Another lesson I really learned was how people treat handicapped people. Some were very rude, would not wait for you to get across, or hold a door for you. Others could not have been kinder and more helpful. I am sorry to say I was one that was often impatient, but not rude. It gave me a new insight and now I will gladly wait on or help someone who is handicapped. I have been there, understand the feelings of helplessness, appreciated the help and generosity, and dealt with the rudeness. A handicapped person does not have a choice in their circumstances. Be kind to them because one day it just might be you.

Fortunately, through all this recovery I had short-term disability through my employer as well as the supplemental insurance I had purchased. Thank goodness I had the foresight and purchased those policies. Unfortunately, on a medical leave of absence my job was only guaranteed for twelve weeks. I had to return to work by then or I would lose my job. The screws were supposed to come out after twelve weeks. The doctor didn't want to release me at that point because I still had to do physical therapy, but I explained to him that without the job I would have no insurance and physical therapy would not happen. He said he just couldn't do it without major restrictions and without me talking to my boss first.

I went in and spoke to the Marshal, asking if there was anything he could do for me, because if I didn't get proper treatment the complications could affect me ever walking again. I also explained that once I was back I would need to leave early three afternoons a week for physical therapy. The Marshal was very kind about it and agreed to make this work for me. In the meantime the other records clerk (there was only two of us) had been terminated back in June so the Animal Control Officer had been filling in. Work had been constantly calling me on the phone regarding how to do this and that. If I could come back they would do whatever was necessary to satisfy the doctor's concerns.

In the middle of August, I went back to Flagstaff and registered as an outpatient to have the screws removed from my leg. I was put under a general anesthesia for the procedure. It was amazing the next day when after the screws had been removed and the Novocain had worn off, there was no more piercing pain. The doctor also gave me the screws as a souvenir. They were huge. One measured two and a half inches long and the other was two and three-quarter inches long and looked like something you could buy at the Ace Hardware store, only they cost a whole lot more. In fact, the brand was Ace and they cost $517.00 each including the one that went through the bone and was discarded.

Finally, that next Monday I returned to work with numerous limitations. I had to use a walker, could not do stairs, could not step up in to the vault room or run the normal daily errands to Town Hall. Everyone was more than helpful in running errands, taking faxes up to dispatch, and getting in the vault for me along with many other details. Normally I would be running up and down the stairs at least a dozen times a day but others had to do it for me.

Two weeks later I went back to Flagstaff and had the stitches removed and graduated to a cane. I had come a long way from being bedridden, but still had a long way to go. After all, I had physical therapy facing me.

Most people don't realize how expensive an injury can cost. Even though I had insurance, the patient's financial responsibility was enormous. The total injury cost over $55,000. That included the ground ambulance, helicopter, hospital charges, the anesthesiologist, physical therapy, prescriptions, weekly blood tests to monitor my clotting time since I was on the blood thinner Coumadin, chest x-rays because I developed pneumonia, a wheelchair, walker, crutches, and a cane. The doctor and helicopter were not in my preferred plan so I had to pay out of network fees, which were more than the 20%. I did reach my deductible and out-of-pocket quickly though, and that definitely helped. That amount of money was only from one injury. Even with the supplemental insurance I still suffered a payroll cut since I was on short-term disability. That made the injury even more expensive.

And again, full cervical spinal stabilization.

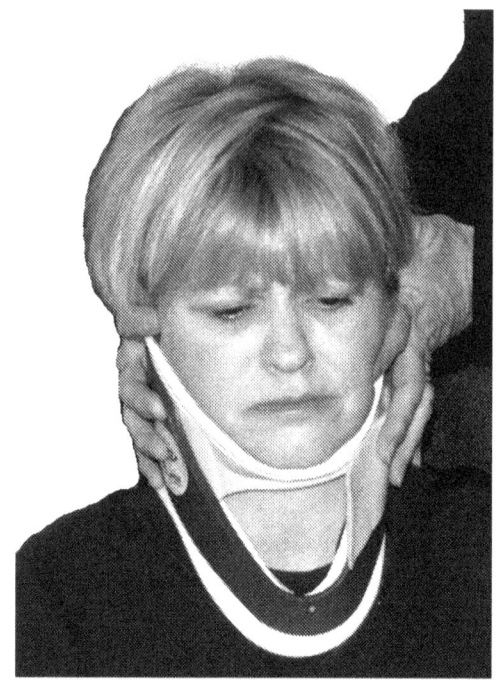

Again, secured on a backboard for transport.

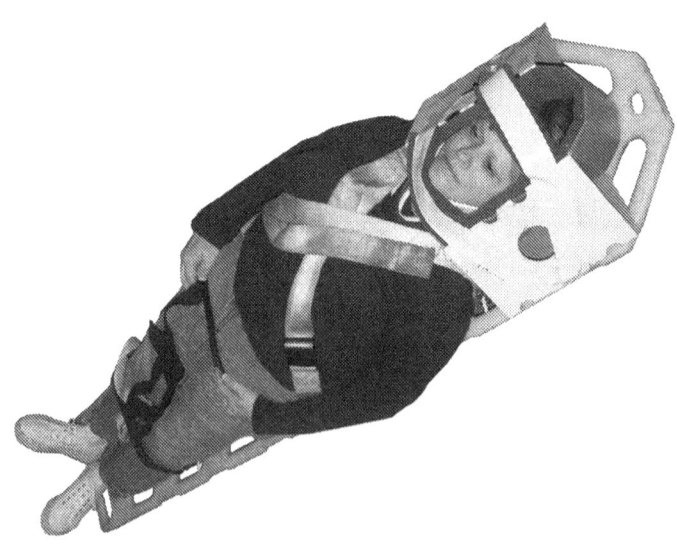

**Transported from camp by ground ambulance
to a landing zone for the helicopter.**

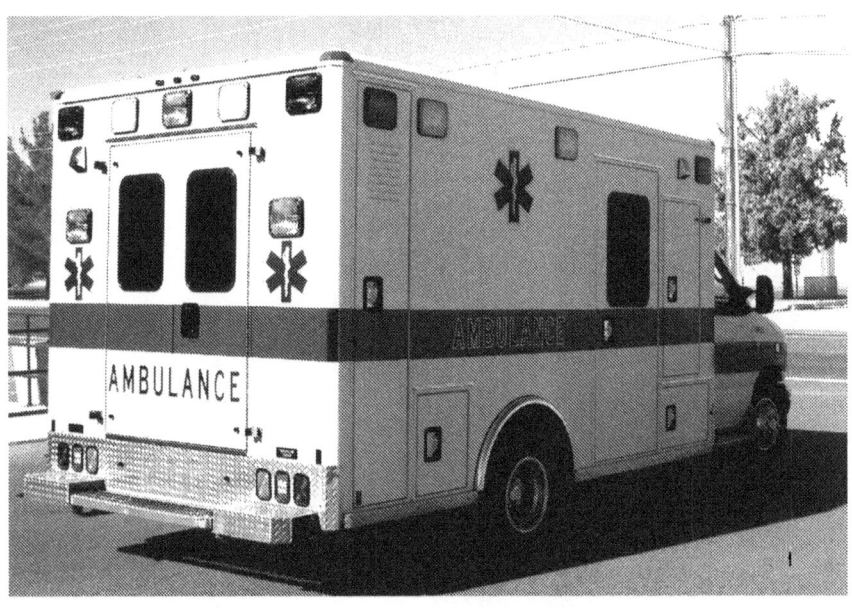

Arriving at Flagstaff Medical Center in a medical helicopter.

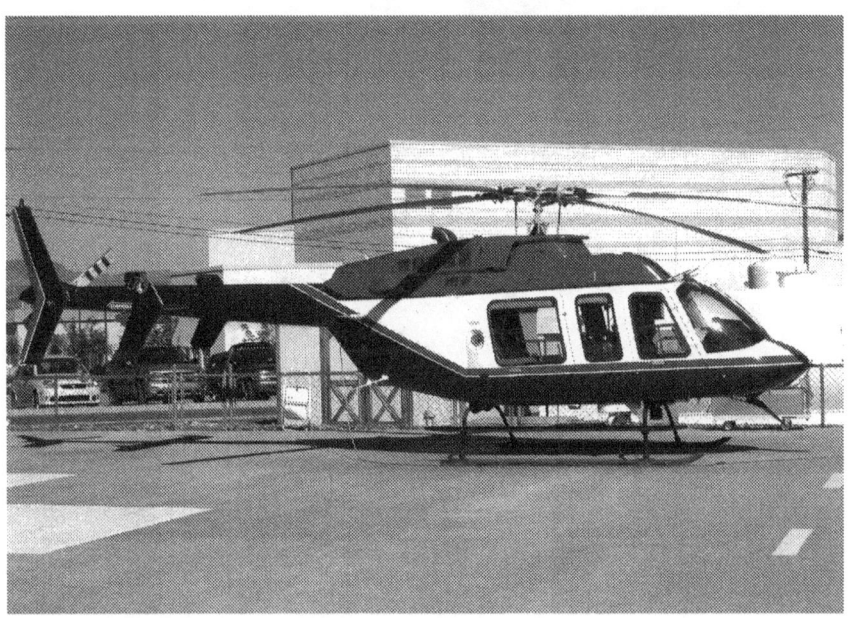

Hinged Knee Immobilizer

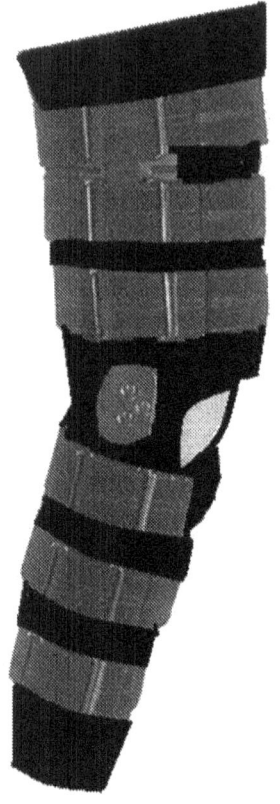

Photo of screws removed.

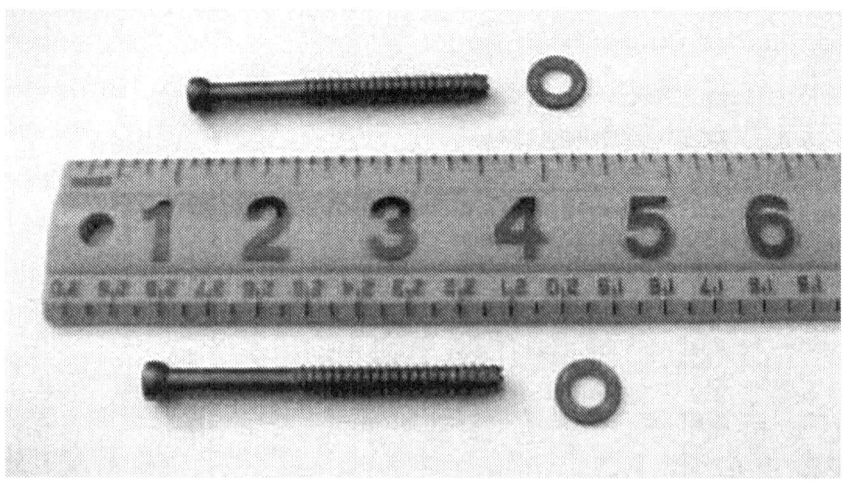

Progress of Mobility

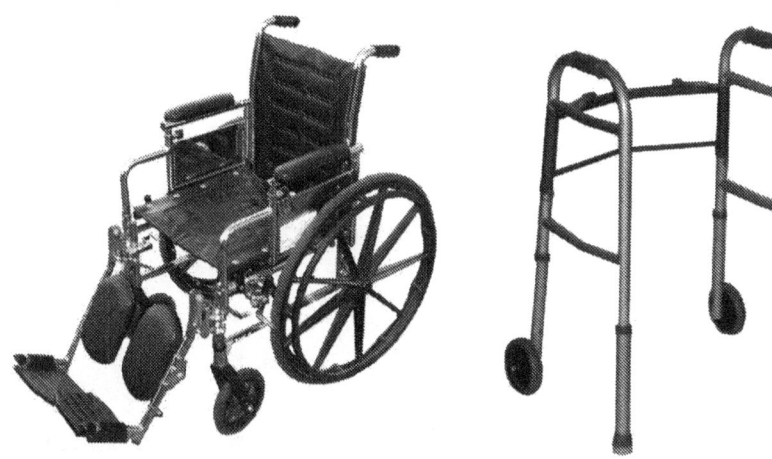

First, a wheelchair.

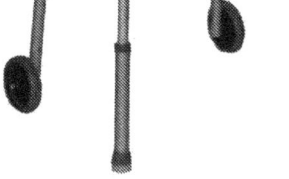

Then a walker.

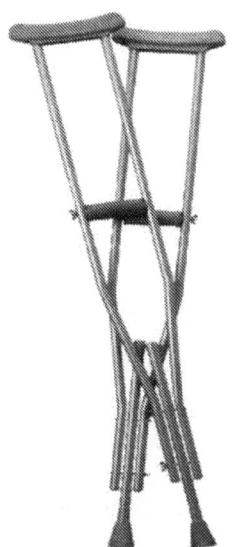

Followed by crutches.

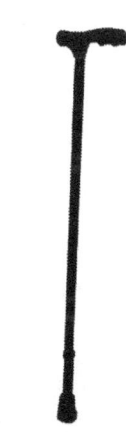

And finally, a cane.

Chapter 14

Beginning in September, I was once again in physical therapy three times a week. I worked through the lunch hour on the days I left work early so I would not lose time or pay. Fortunately, therapy was in Cottonwood, where I lived, so once I was done I went home. I scheduled my appointments so that I got out at the same time I would have gotten off work. And having learned from the past, I took pain medication about 45 minutes before my hour long therapy began.

If I thought therapy was painful with the knee recovery, it was pure hell with the leg. It was absolutely excruciating, plain and simple. At times I thought I would die before I was finished. All I wanted to do was quit, go home, and crawl in bed. The only thing that kept me going was that I didn't want to be back in a wheelchair. That was my motivation. But once therapy was finished for the day, I did go home and crawl into bed.

In the beginning my sessions began with electrical stimulation followed by walking very slowly on the treadmill. As time went by I was able to increase the speed and distance as well as endurance. As therapy progressed I also used an air bicycle, a leg weight machine, scooted across the floor on an office chair with wheels, did stepping exercises and walked a line like they would do for a sobriety test. Each session through the very last one ended with an icepack for 20 minutes.

At home I had ankle weights and did certain exercises to strengthen the leg. I also had an office chair at my computer desk so I did that exercise going back and forth down the hall. Since I owned a treadmill I used that only on the weekends.

The therapist explained to me the importance of doing home exercises, but that with the type of injury I had, I could also overdue it and had to be careful. Limits were place on what I did and the number of repetitions.

Every several weeks I had to go to Flagstaff and the doctor would examine my leg and check on my progress. Depending on how the leg was feeling, he had me use either crutches or the cane. I had graduated to a cane earlier but he felt crutches should be used if I had any weakness. He didn't want me going down. I was to use my judgment in that decision.

Each visit included a medical update on my physical limitations and restrictions for both home and work. That update was placed in my personnel file both at the Marshal's Office and at Town Hall. Basically the restrictions and limitations never changed. I was not to use a ladder, stoop, kneel, crawl, or lift over eight pounds. I could use stairs with caution.

Because of the fracture, my baths had been replaced with showers. On Super Bowl Sunday 2004, after Randy went to the grocery store, I decided that I would try taking a bath. I had been putting weight on the leg and bending the knee for sometime and felt I could accomplish this. I was tired of showers and just craved soaking in a tub full of hot water and bubble bath. So I filled the tub and worked my way down. And I did it! I was actually able to get down in the bathtub with all that hot, bubble bath. I thought I had died and gone to heaven. I had the water all the way up to my neck and thoroughly enjoyed the luxury that I never thought would happen again. When Randy arrived back home I hollered to him that I was in heaven or as close to it as I could be. Finally, after an hour of soaking, looking like a prune, and having used up all the hot water (as the water cooled I drained it and kept adding more hot water), it was time to try getting out. After the water drained, I got on all fours and was able to get out of the tub. Life was good; I was back to taking baths.

I noticed during this time of year I was in mild to moderate pain quite a bit. I was sitting at my desk too much and needed to move around more. I was also falling more frequently. Fortunately, it usually happened when I was alone; however it did leave me with bruises or broken ribs. I mentioned it to the doctor who had treated me for the leg fracture and he said that my left knee was going out but he didn't want to do a replacement surgery yet. The osteoporosis was as much to blame. The muscles and bones were weak and if I continued to fall I would need to use a cane all the time. So now I knew why I my leg gave out causing me to fall so much.

Physical therapy continued until late February 2004. At that time the doctor released me from his care and physical therapy. My range of motion had reached its full potential of 115 degrees. He felt it would not go beyond that. I was officially healed the best I would be. The doctor stressed the importance of my lifetime restrictions. Still no stooping, kneeling, crawling, ladders, lifting over eight pounds, long periods of sitting or standing, or anything else that could cause stress on the knees, hips, back, neck, or spine. I was not to camp anymore because of rough terrain. The chances of falling and getting injured were too high. That meant I needed to resign from Search and Rescue as well. It was hard to believe that part of my life was over. As I walked out to my vehicle and started the drive back to Cottonwood from Flagstaff, I wondered when I would have my next major injury and what the results would be.

Physical Therapy Exercises

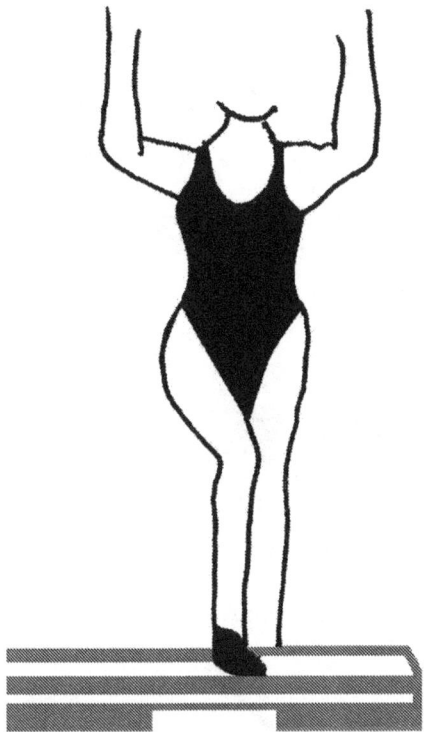

Step Exercises

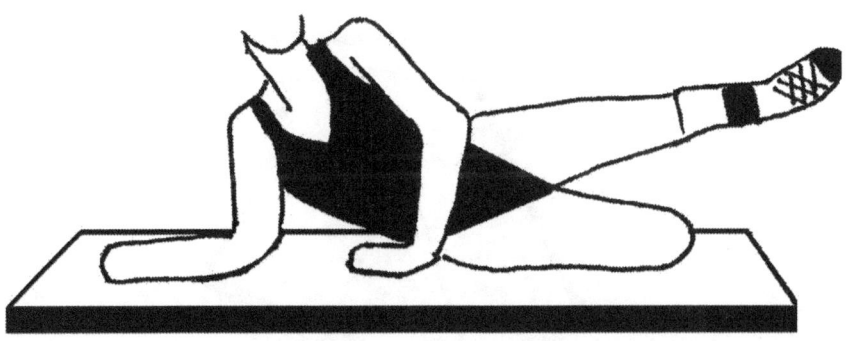

Leg Lifts with Ankle Weights

Physical Therapy Exercises Continued

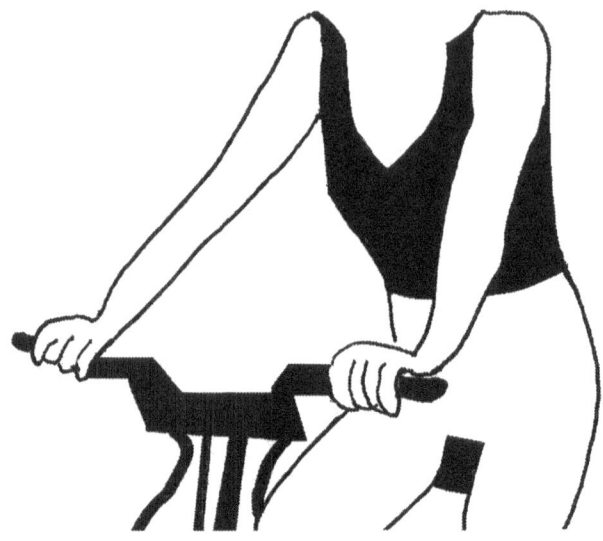

Stationary Bicycle

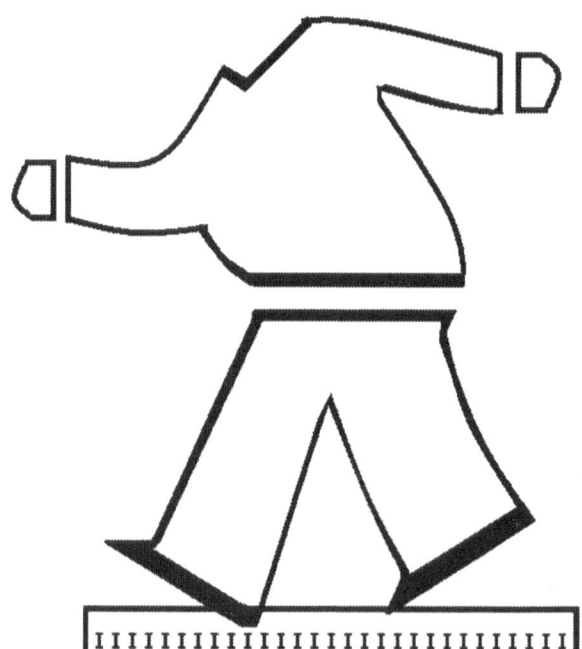

Straight Line Walk

Chapter 15

I suppose it was around late March of 2004, that I began having hot flashes and memory problems. I was also feeling quite depressed, would get upset at the drop of a hat, and start crying. I also had a stomach that would not go down no matter what I did or did not eat, or however much I exercised. As time went by, all of it just seemed to get worse.

There had been a lot of stress at work. The Marshal had been placed on administrative leave in January and one of the Sergeants' had been asked by the Town Manager to be the Interim Marshal until a hearing and decision was completed. I was the secretary to the Marshal and now Administrative Assistant to the Interim Marshal. To make things harder on our department, in April we lost a deputy in a tragic accident. We had just hired a new records clerk and I was in the process of training her. Lots of changes were going on at work. I would go into the bathroom to cry but eventually I just started doing it out in the open. Each night when I went home I was so tired and depressed that I had no desire to think about preparing dinner. I was also having a lot of back and hip pain, which did not help. All I wanted to do was take a bath and go to bed, which is usually what I did.

The emotional roller coaster, hot flashes, and pain finally became so bad, affecting me both at home and at work that I went to see my family internist. I was stunned with the diagnosis. I was going through both depression and menopause. The pain was caused by the osteoporosis. Apparently the depression had been building up for years — possibly as far back as when my ex-husband and I separated. I thought I had done quite well with it, but apparently not. That would explain some of the uncontrollable crying spells. As for the menopause, I told the doctor I went through it 24 years ago because of the total hysterectomy. I was told that because I was nearing my 50's, my body still thought it needed to go through it. My reply was that it wasn't fair to have to go through it twice!

Since hormone replacement therapy was not an option for me, I would have to work through menopause, but the depression was treatable. I began taking Effexor and was monitored closely in the beginning. If the Effexor worked, the doctor thought after a couple of years I would probably wean off of it, but first it had to work. After getting to the maximum dosage around six weeks after beginning the medication, my husband and I began to notice big changes. I no longer was crying as much as I did and was able to cope with situations better. As time continued to go by, the crying ceased completely. I was not bothered by things like I used to be and life seemed to be improving. One side effect of Effexor is uncontrollable weight loss, to the point of anorexia. However I only lost about eight pounds. After having been on Effexor for six months, it was hard to remember how difficult that time in my life was.

In August, a permanent new Marshal was hired. As with any new leader there were again numerous changes. Some of those changes were subtler than others. More stress was added to the work life but I continued on. Supervisor positions changed and new policies were implemented as old ones went out the window. Some changes were for the better and some would require sitting back and waiting to see if they were worth it.

As the new Marshal settled in, he began to review everyone's personnel file. In November, when he finally got to mine, I was questioned about my physical restrictions and limitations. I explained to him I suffered from severe osteoporosis and that there were certain things I was and was not allowed to do. The Marshal said he needed a new written medical update from my doctor for my file since the one in my case file was over a year old (that was from the date I returned back to work — not from having finished physical therapy).

I made an appointment with my local internist and I was told I needed a new bone mineral density test done since it had been so long since the last one. At least having insurance this time made it easier. The test was scheduled for December 15, 2004 at my doctor's office in Sedona, Arizona. They had a new bone density-scanning machine and that would save me the drive to Scottsdale. On December 23, I went back for my test results. I knew they would be bad but had no idea my life was to come crashing down on me. My spine had a T-Score of −4.1 and a Z-Score of −3.4. My hip T-Score was −3.6 and my Z-Score −2.4. I was in very serious trouble. I was now 49 with the bones of someone who would be in their 90's. I needed to cease working because I had a serious medical disability. I was too much of a risk to any employer and to myself — especially since the next fall could be the one that made me a paraplegic or quadriplegic and put me in the wheelchair.

I asked the doctor if I had some time to get things in order. I needed to check in to short-term and long-term disability and find out all the qualifications. I knew short- term would not be a problem since I had used it in 2003, but long-term was new to me. I didn't know how to go about it; if I had worked long enough to qualify and what was required for acceptance. My plan was to work through February or March as I researched everything and basically got my "ducks in a row."

Since it was only two days until Christmas and the next day was a paid holiday because Christmas was on Saturday, I had time to think clearly at home while discussing everything with my husband. I had already called him as I was driving back home from the doctor. Being the romantic that he is, he arrived home with a dozen red roses for me. Then he just held me while I cried and cried, telling me we would get through this.

One good thing was that as long as I was on short-term disability, my employer had to maintain my current medical, dental, and vision insurance. They also had to pay for all of my supplemental insurance policies and I was not required to reimburse them. I had learned this the last time I was on short-term disability when I had the tibial plateau fracture in 2003.

Insurance had been so important, especially all the supplemental policies that I owned. I had to find out what the process was for maintaining them once I was no longer employed. I knew that the payments would change from my employer making the payments after deducting it from my salary, to an automatic debit from my checking account, but I didn't know how long that took to go in to effect and I couldn't afford a lapse in any of the policies because any lapse would cause me to lose them. After the holidays were over I would look into long-term disability.

The Spine

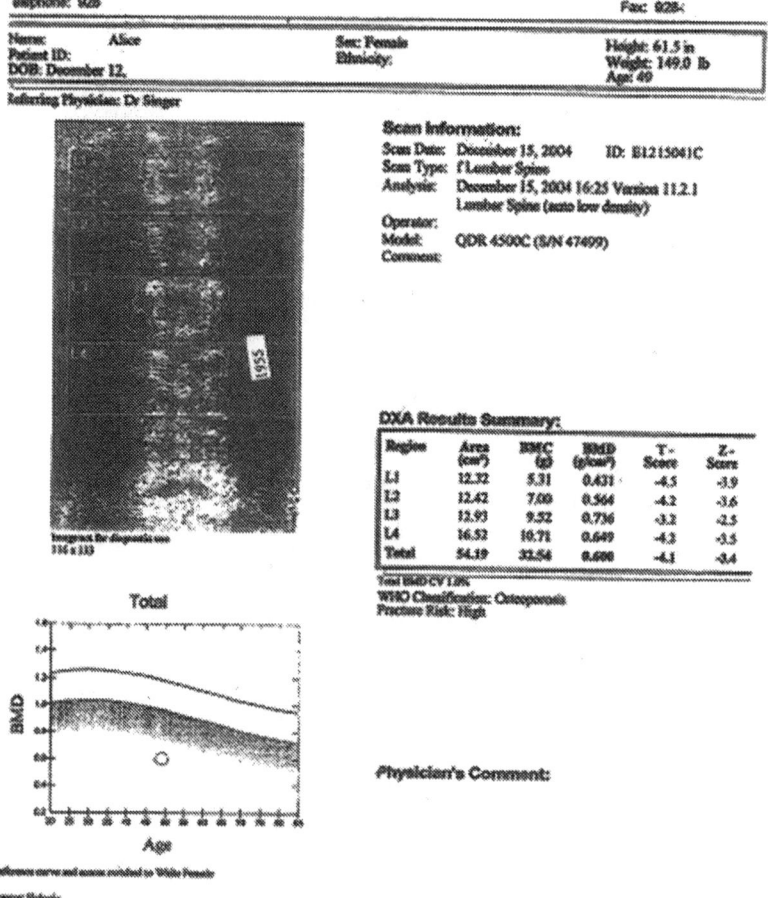

3700 West Hwy. 89A
Sedona, AZ 86336

Telephone: 928-   Fax: 928-

Name: Alice
Patient ID:
DOB: December 12,
Referring Physician: Dr Singer

Sex: Female
Ethnicity:

Height: 61.5 in
Weight: 149.0 lb
Age: 49

Scan Information:
Scan Date: December 15, 2004   ID: B1215041C
Scan Type: f Lumbar Spine
Analysis: December 15, 2004 16:25 Version 11.2.1
Lumbar Spine (auto low density)
Operator:
Model: QDR 4500C (S/N 47499)
Comment:

DXA Results Summary:

Region	Area (cm²)	BMC (g)	BMD (g/cm²)	T-Score	Z-Score
L1	12.32	5.31	0.431	-4.5	-3.9
L2	12.42	7.09	0.564	-4.2	-3.6
L3	13.93	9.52	0.736	-3.2	-2.5
L4	16.52	10.71	0.649	-4.3	-3.5
Total	54.19	32.54	0.606	-4.1	-3.4

Total BMD CV 1.0%
WHO Classification: Osteoporosis
Fracture Risk: High

Total

Physician's Comment:

BMD

Age

Reference curve and scores matched to White Female

Source: Hologic

Bone Mineral Density Test Results.

Right Hip

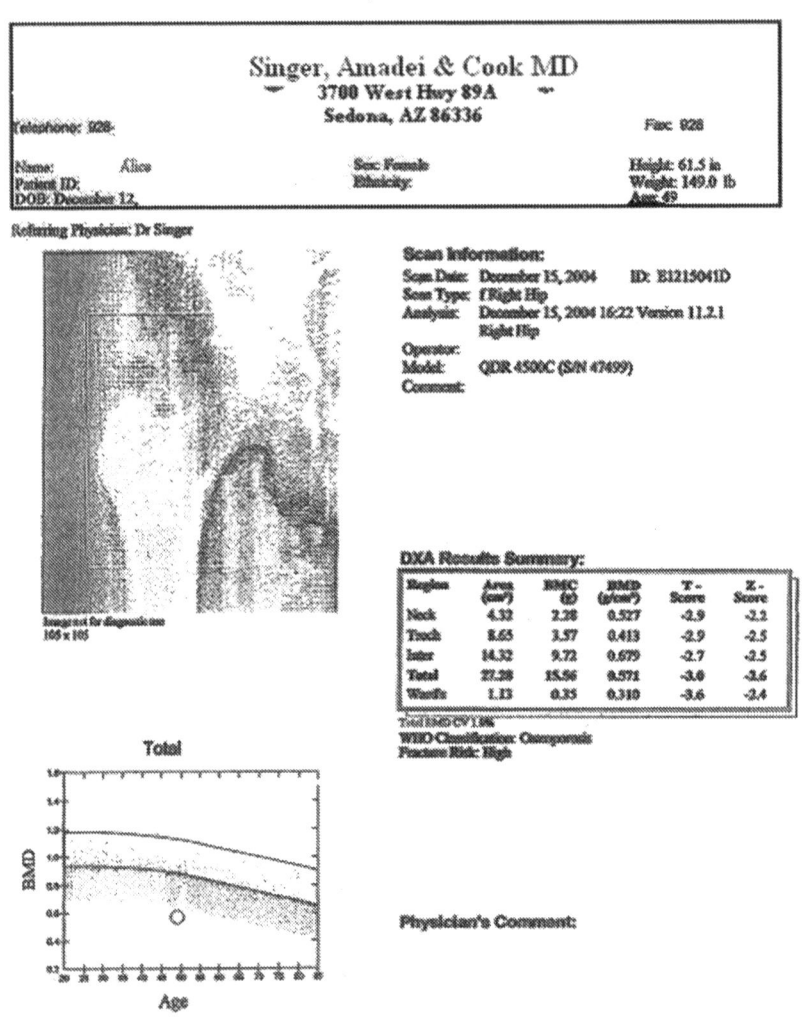

Bone Mineral Density Test Results.

Chapter 16

On December 28, 2004, the unthinkable happened. I fell at work while several people were in the office with me. I hurt my lower back, neck, and left hip. This time I couldn't get up and keep it a secret. An ambulance was immediately dispatched and the Marshal had someone notify my husband that I was being transported to the hospital in Cottonwood. The paramedic gave me morphine for the pain and I couldn't stop crying, both because of the pain and because I knew my days at work were over. That was officially my last day at work. Short-term disability began when I fell to the ground. So much for waiting until February or March in the New Year; obviously I was not in control of my own life.

Once at the hospital I went through numerous x-rays. Over 35 x-rays were taken of my spine, hip, and neck to ensure there was no major damage considering my medical history. Thank God, nothing was broken. I did bruise and was banged up from twisting and turning as I fell so that nothing would break. Its amazing in those split seconds before I hit the ground, how well I had consciously trained myself to sprain or bruise something by twisting and turning to avoid a fracture; I guess it comes from years of falls. I was released from the emergency room with strong pain medication and told to contact my doctor the beginning of that next week.

I immediately followed up with my doctor who also discussed a new medication called, Forteo that was available and actually helped to build bone back up. In January of 2005, I attended a class held by a representative of the manufacturing company for this new drug. The purpose of the class was to learn about osteoporosis, the medication to be used, its attributes, any of its complications or reactions, and how to inject it into my abdomen on a daily basis. This form of therapy would last for a maximum period of two years if there were no side affects or complications. Being sensitive to so many medications I was quite apprehensive but truly hoped for the best. This was my last chance for a medication to have a positive result; and I needed it desperately.

I took the class with five other individuals, all with varying degrees of osteoporosis. It really hit me hard to be the youngest one participating in the class with the worst test results. A woman almost 90 years old was there and her results weren't nearly as bad as mine. That was definitely another reality check for me. I needed to stick with this program no matter what. I prayed I would be able to tolerate the medicine. Even if there were complications or reactions to it, as long as it was tolerable and without dangerous risks I would do it. I committed myself to that plan.

When the time came to learn how to give myself a shot in the abdomen, it was very difficult for me. The medication comes in a pen type syringe with a pre-measured dosage that is good for 28 days. I learned how to prep the pen, tap for air bubbles, and then release a small amount to guarantee the needle was not clogged or defective. Then I was to inject the full dosage into my abdomen. Well, you have no idea how many times I counted to ten and could not convince myself to get it in. Finally, after a self-lecture that told myself, "That's fine. You don't need to do this. Just get the wheelchair out and polished up, because that was where you're headed." I counted, "One, two, three," and in it went. My phobia was over and I knew I could do it.

Once at home, my husband stood in disbelief as I gave myself the injection. Being a medic, it didn't bother him at all and he could have done it for me. But, as he watched me inject the medication into myself he said he never thought he would see the day that I would give myself a shot. I had come a long way. I told him I wanted to walk with my grandchildren; not have them ride in my lap. Any little thing of special meaning that I would no longer be able to do gave me the incentive to keep doing it each day. If that is what it took to do it then so be it. Whatever helped me get through that beginning period was all that mattered. This medication would cost $1300 per month without insurance, so I was grateful beyond measure that I had insurance because it would only cost me $137 per month for two years.

Applying for short-term disability would last for a period of six months and it was not without diversions and obstacles. Numerous forms needed to be completed by my doctor, employer, and myself on a continuing basis. The forms were then mailed to the proper insurance companies for acceptance and payments. With the short-term insurance provided by my employer, I would receive 60% of my salary after taxes every two weeks for six months. At the end of that six-month period my income would cease and all insurance policies were my responsibility.

At the end of short-term disability I had the option of purchasing the medical, dental, and vision polices provided by my employer. After careful deliberation, my husband and I decided to purchase a Cobra Plan for medical insurance only. It would cost over $400 each month, but it was a policy I couldn't afford to be without. There was no way I could afford the full cost of the Forteo and that didn't take in to account my other monthly prescriptions as well as any emergencies that could happen in the future or if I broke another bone.

So while I was still on short-term I went to the dentist and had everything checked out and taken care of. I also visited my eye doctor and learned I needed a new prescription for glasses. I had a physical and tried to take care of anything else during that first six-month period.

In March of 2005, I met with my doctor, an endocrinologist at the Mayo Clinic in Scottsdale, Arizona. I took with me the results of the bone mineral density tests that were done in December of 2004, by my primary care doctor in Sedona, Arizona. My doctor was very direct saying said that in addition to the daily Forteo injections I was giving myself in the abdomen, I needed to take 1500 milligrams of calcium (five hundred milligrams three times daily). I needed to double or triple the 400 units of vitamin D that I had been taking daily. Without the increased dosages of calcium and vitamin D, the Forteo would be worthless and I would see no change.

At the time, Forteo was the only drug proven to not only stop bone loss, but also actually rebuild bone. It can, however, only be taken for maximum of two years. In my case, since there is so much bone loss, any new growth would be a surprise. It would never change the fact that I have severe osteoporosis. Hopefully, though, the Forteo might prevent any further loss of bone mass. With the amount of bone loss I have suffered, the medication would never get me to a good score, but at least it might not get any worse.

As a result of the severe osteoporosis I had shrunk again, losing one and a half inches. On my first visit to the Mayo Clinic in 1991, I measured five feet two inches tall. In 1995, I was five feet one and one-half inches. In March 2005, I came in at just five feet tall.

I was told that for the rest of my life I would need to use either a cane or walker to assist me in hopes of preventing further falls. I own a treadmill and could use it with caution as long as I held on and did not fall. Again, the importance of daily swimming was stressed. I wasn't to lift over five pounds at any time for the rest of my life. If I continued to fall and had not become paralyzed I could still end up in a wheelchair to prevent paralysis from happening. It would depend on doing the necessary exercises and how much muscle strength I could build up to protect the bones in a fall.

Extensive blood work was done. I was told to call back in four days for the results. If all the test results looked good, the doctor didn't need to see me for a year. If any of the tests came back questionable, then I would have to arrange another appointment with him. In the meantime, he would consult with my primary care doctor who would oversee me locally. Fortunately, I later learned the blood work came back without any major problems, so that was one less matter to deal with.

There was nothing else that could be done for me. The doctor stressed the importance of following all of the suggestions given to me. The next fall could be the one that made me a paraplegic or quadriplegic.

Then, early in April 2005, I fell in the living room at home. As I went down I grabbed a floor lamp nearby in hopes of catching the fall. I was actually trying to reach for a moderately large secretary but got the lamp instead. Later, my husband said it was a good thing I didn't get hold of the secretary because it probably would have landed on top of me. Once I went down, both the cat and dog were right there with me acting very concerned.

It was a wonderfully pleasant spring day. All of the windows and screen doors were open for fresh air, and there I lay on the floor. My husband had just gone back to work about 45 minutes earlier after having been home for lunch. After lying on the floor for approximately 20 to 30 minutes I heard voices next door, so I started yelling for help. It took about 15 minutes before someone heard me. Apparently, the neighbor next door was having a yard sale and a customer heard me. They came over, called 911 and my husband, locked the cat up, put the dog in the back yard, and moved the broken lamp I had taken to the floor with me. Once the Fire Department and ambulance arrived I was placed in that never-ending cervical collar and trussed up on a backboard like a turkey ready for roasting. While I was being "packaged" for transport, one of the paramedics suggested I talk to my doctor about an alert button, since I am home alone. If I fell I could push it and emergency personnel would automatically be dispatched to my house.

At the hospital and after many x-rays, the emergency room doctor gave me the good news that nothing was broken. I was, however, already beginning to bruise up. He said the worst pain would be on day two or three. A prescription for pain medication was given to me prior to discharge. The doctor also suggested the alert button and to follow up with my doctor. Three and a half hours later I was on my way home to nurse my aching body.

Regarding long-term disability, I was eligible to apply through the State of Arizona. Whether I was accepted would depend on the various doctors' reports regarding the severity of my osteoporosis. After being on short-term for six months I could apply for long-term disability. If I was accepted, and since it could take up to six months to start, payment eligibility would begin the day short-term ended. If I was approved the monthly payment would be 66% of my gross salary tax-free. All my husband and I had to do was figure out how to get by for up to six months before receiving back pay. Then on a set day each month, the appropriate funds would automatically be deposited in to my checking account if I were eligible.

As of July 4, 2005, short-term disability was officially over. The application and medical release forms had been sent to the insurance company responsible for long- term disability. I did have to make a trip to Social Security to show that I didn't have enough quarters in to qualify for medical disability or Medicare. If I had qualified that amount would have been deducted from long-term amount that I would be entitled to monthly.

All the doctors who have treated my fractures over the years had been requested to send documentation to help in the decision process. Fortunately, I had also kept copies of major injuries. As it turned out I did have to send some of my copies because one doctor had moved from Flagstaff to Phoenix.

In the beginning of August, I learned my claim for long-term disability had been approved pending verification from my employer. After speaking to the Human Resource Office of my former employer, they said as soon as the paperwork arrived, they would sign and mail it back as soon as possible. It only took five weeks for a decision, not the dreaded six months. I figured it would take at least another month to get the payment arrangement in place and working smoothly. But the first deposit was made in two weeks.

Chapter 17

As I mentioned early on in the book, osteoporosis — the most common skeletal disorder in our country — does not discriminate. It affects the young and the old, men and women. Men can get the hip and other fractures that come with osteoporosis just as women do. Osteoporosis related fractures or injuries are just as debilitating and painful to men. So I felt it was only appropriate to dedicate a chapter to men.

If detected before significant bone loss has occurred, osteoporosis can be treated effectively. A medical work-up to diagnose osteoporosis, would include blood tests, complete medical history, urine tests, and x-rays. The bone mineral density test BMD) can be used to detect low bone density, predict risk for future fractures, diagnose osteoporosis, and monitor treatments.

Doctors, however, are unsure how to interpret the results of a BMD test in men. According to the National Institute of Health, it's not known if the guidelines used to diagnose osteoporosis or low bone mass in women are also appropriate for men. Still, it is a good start.

A low bone mineral density and excessive bone loss are the two major contributing factors resulting in some type of fracture among men. In men there are two types of osteoporosis: primary and secondary, says the National Institute of Health.

In the cases of primary osteoporosis, the condition is caused by age-related bone loss (which has been referred to as senile osteoporosis) or the cause is unknown (known as (idiopathic osteoporosis). The term idiopathic osteoporosis is used for men under the age of 70; over age 70, age-related bone loss (senile osteoporosis) is assumed to be the cause.

In cases of secondary osteoporosis, the loss of bone mass is caused by certain lifestyles, behaviors, diseases, or medication. The most common causes include low levels of testosterone, alcohol abuse, smoking, gastrointestinal disease, hypercalciuria (excessive quantities of calcium in the urine), and immobilization.

Hypogonadism refers to abnormally low levels of hormones. It's well known that loss of estrogen causes osteoporosis. Just as pre- and post-menopausal women experience a decrease in estrogen; in men reduced levels of the sex hormones may also cause osteoporosis. Since testosterone affects the levels of estrogen in men, men with lower estrogen levels lose bone mass faster than men with higher estrogen levels. Most men do not experience the sudden hormonal change that women do as a result of menopause. But it can happen. According to the National Institute of Health, it is estimated that up to 30% of men who experience osteoporotic vertebral fractures have low testosterone levels. Certain medications like steroids, cancer treatment (especially for prostate cancer) and many other factors can be responsible for sudden changes in the testosterone level.

Because, however, the majority of men have larger and stronger bones than women, bone loss usually begins later and advances slower than the female gender. But by the ages 65 to 70, men and women lose bone mass at the same rate, and the absorption of calcium, an essential nutrient for bone health throughout life, decreases in both sexes. Osteoporosis in men has become more of an important public issue in the last few years. Definitely information is needed about the causes and treatment of osteoporosis according to the NIH. The results of such studies will help physicians better understand how to prevent, manage, and treat men with osteoporosis.

Studies have also shown that a large number of men experiencing specific hormone abnormalities have also been linked to excessive drinking and/or smoking. As I mentioned in Chapter One, alcohol affects the body's ability to absorb calcium, and smoking decreases calcium absorption in the intestines.

Several nutrients, including amino acids, calcium, magnesium, phosphorus, and vitamins D and K, are important for bone health. Diseases of the stomach and intestines can lead to bone disease when they impair absorption of these nutrients. Treatment for bone loss in this case may include supplementation of the poorly absorbed nutrient(s) says the NIH.

Affecting both men and women, losing too much calcium in the urine (Hypercalciuria) will also cause bone loss. This happens twice as much in men as it does in women. By talking to your doctor however, treatment options are available if necessary after the proper testing.

Immobilization according to the National Institute of Health is another major factor. Weight-bearing exercise is essential for maintaining bones; without it bone density may rapidly decline. Prolonged bed rest (following fractures, surgery, spinal cord injuries, or illness) or immobilization of some part of the body often results in significant bone loss. Therefore it's crucial to resume weight-bearing exercises as soon as possible after a prolonged bed rest. Dancing, jogging, walking, and weight lifting are a few examples of weight-bearing exercises.

Some of the risk factors for men are the same as in women and include family history (osteoporosis is hereditary), consuming excessive amounts of alcohol, inactivity, lack of weight-bearing exercise, a lean body build, a diet of high protein and low calcium intake, low vitamin

D intake (vitamin D is crucial in the absorption of calcium), certain medications (like thyroid replacement and steroids are just a couple), race (Caucasians and Asians are most susceptible), low testosterone levels, premature graying hair, and smoking. Age is one risk factor that cannot be controlled; the older a person is, the greater the risk of getting osteoporosis.

Osteoporosis was always considered a "woman's disease" and somehow men were overlooked. But by the end of the year 2005, the number of hip fractures among men equaled the number of women with hip fractures. Men are three times more likely then women to suffer complications or death as a result of a hip fracture during the first year. The National Institute of Health claims that men who sustain hip fractures are more likely to die than women. Half of all men who suffer from a hip fracture are discharged to a nursing home. 79% percent of those who survive for one year after a hip fracture still live in nursing homes or intermediate care facilities.

Men also suffer fractures to the vertebrae. According to the National Institute of Health- Osteoporosis and Related Bone Diseases, symptomatic vertebral (spine) fractures occur about half as often in men as in women, and with those fractures, men are just as prone to end up with the stooped posture (hunch back) as women are. Rib and wrist fractures are also just as likely to occur in men as they do in women. Just as in women, fractures in men can be disabling. Mobility may require the assistance of a cane, walker, wheelchair, or even an electric scooter.

Certain medications have been approved for men. That is why it's important to consult a doctor if there are any concerns. The doctor may want to monitor the male patient for various reasons including but not limited to bone density, calcium intake as well as vitamin D, exercise, nutrition, and testosterone levels.

Recognize and treat any health problem that can affect bone health. Avoid smoking; refraining from excessive alcoholic beverages, engaging in a regular routine of weight bearing exercises and having a calcium rich balanced diet will decrease some of the risks of acquiring osteoporosis. The National Institute of Health recommends getting enough daily calcium. Men over fifty need 1200 mg of calcium daily, but consult your doctor for accuracy as he reviews your personal health history. By adding fortified orange juice and cereals, eating lots of leafy green vegetables and low-in fat dairy products like cheese, ice cream, milk and yogurt to your diet is a good start. The NIH says dietary vitamin D intake should be at least 400 IU but not more than 800 IU per day. 400 IU is the amount found in one quart of fortified milk and most multivitamins.

Recommendations for Calcium and Vitamin D Intake in Men[18]

Age	Calcium (mg)	Vitamin D (IU)
19-30	1,000	-----
31-50	1,000	200
51-70	1,200	400
70+	1,200	600
Upper Limit	2,500	2,500

The NIH also stresses the importance of regular weight-bearing exercises, such as dancing, walking, jogging, racquet sports, stair climbing, tennis, weight training, and using resistance machines. These

---

[18] This chart is courtesy of the National Institute of Health - Osteoporosis and Related Bone Disease

exercises may strengthen your bones. This may help your balance and reduce the risks of falls, thus reducing the chance of a fracture. Preventing falls will reduce the chances of a fracture plus you will feel healthier and more confident. Remember it's important to consult your doctor prior to beginning any new exercise program.

It's just as important for men to consult their doctor as it is for women. Once bone is lost, it cannot be completely replaced. As bone mass is lost, bone fragility rises and there is more likelihood of experiencing a fracture. But with early detection before major bone loss occurs, a proper therapy treatment can slow down or even prevent osteoporosis. Telling your doctor about any change in posture, loss in height, unusual fractures, or back pain can help the doctor in his evaluation. The bone mineral density test can also show if there is a risk for fractures in the future. Make a list to take with you regarding any concerns. Be totally honest when answering questions.

Today, many men with osteoporosis are being prescribed most of the same medications that women receive. Their doctor can determine the best medication and route of therapy depending on the patient and his complete medical history.

Yet even with all this knowledge and understanding, men still view osteoporosis as a "woman's disease" and do not think of themselves as having osteoporosis. They may only find out that they have it when seeking medical attention for a fracture. There is still so much to learn about osteoporosis, both in men and women. That is why it's so important to see your doctor before you are diagnosed with osteoporosis. Learn your options early to prevent or slow down the "silent disease." Accept your doctor's suggestions with an open mind and make a commitment to yourself to follow through with his recommendations. Your health, your future, your bones, and your family depend on it.

Chapter 18

Preventative measures are just as important to help slow down the development of osteoporosis or in living with it. If someone has been diagnosed with the disease, it's important that they take it seriously. To take the diagnosis of osteoporosis lightly and not adhere to the limitations given by the doctor can result in increased bone loss or even serious fractures.

The United States Food and Drug Administration claims changing attitudes and improving technology are brightening the outlook for people with osteoporosis. Nowadays, many women live thirty years or more after menopause. And improving the quality of life has become an important health care goal. Although some bone loss is expected as people age, osteoporosis is no longer viewed as an inevitable consequence of aging. Diagnosis and treatment need no longer wait until bones break.

The FDA sys that there is no cure or proven preventative treatment for osteoporosis, but the onset can be delayed and the severity diminished. Most important, early intervention can help prevent devastating fractures. The Food and Drug Administration has revised labeling on foods and supplements to provide valuable information about the level of nutrients that help build and maintain strong bones.

Treatment options are expanding, so physicians and patients have more options available to them. Under FDA guidelines, drugs to treat osteoporosis must be shown to preserve or increase bone mass and maintain bone quality in order to reduce the risk of fractures. Your doctor can discuss these options with you for your particular medical history.

But drugs are not enough. Calcium intake is critical, but calcium alone can't build bones. Vitamin D is needed to help the body absorb the calcium. Good sources of calcium include low-fat dairy products such as cheese, milk, ice cream, and yogurt. Leafy vegetables like broccoli and spinach, and certain seafood like sardines and salmon also contain calcium. Calcium fortified foods like breads, cereals, and orange juice are just as valuable in the daily diet.

A good habit of weight-bearing exercises also helps maintain strong bones. Depending on your interest there are many choices that include hiking, jogging, stair climbing, tennis, walking, and weight lifting.

Not smoking is very important as it affects the absorption of calcium. If you enjoy alcoholic beverages, do it in moderation.

Falls can be serious at any age, and breaking bones after a fall becomes more likely as a person ages. A simple fall can change your life. I have experienced that myself. After my tibial plateau fracture of the right leg, it never regained its full mobility. Suffering from osteoporosis, a minor fall can become a major injury.

If you are a sufferer of osteoporosis try to make your home more "fall safe." When mopping floors give them plenty of time to dry. Try not to have slippery floors and keep them free of clutter. Wear shoes or slippers with rubber soles. Wearing only socks can cause you to slip on a slick floor. Tack down carpets and throw rugs. Have your vision and hearing checked out. Small changes can make a difference in your safety. If your home has stairs be sure to have handrails and use them when going up and down the stairs. Also make sure the stairs have decent lighting. Leave a night light on while sleeping or have a flashlight nearby. Do not attempt to walk in the dark without some type of light. That is a sure way to trip and fall. When going out, use a cane if necessary. If you live in snow country try not to go out and avoid icy patches if you must be out in adverse weather conditions. Do not rush, take your time, and be safe. Use non- skid mats in the shower or tub and a non-skid rug to step out on to. Keep electrical cords out of the path of traffic.

The NIH says that people are unaware that there is often a link between the broken bone and osteoporosis, a silent disease in which there is a gradual loss of bone tissue or bone density that makes bones so fragile they break under the slightest strain. Because osteoporosis progresses without symptoms, falls are especially dangerous for people who are unaware that they have a low bone density. If the patient and the physician fail to connect the broken bone to osteoporosis, the chances to make a diagnosis with a bone density test and begin prevention or a treatment program is lost. Bone loss continues until another bone breaks.

And this is exactly what happened to me. As I mentioned in Chapter 5, I had been experiencing a number of rib fractures while living in the town of Williams. I also had a fractured right leg. I mentioned too, that the doctor had not picked up on the signs of osteoporosis. As for me, I was clueless at that time. If my doctor had known the warning signs, maybe I would not be as bad off as I am now.

Several factors can lead to falls. Loss of footing, or loss of traction are common causes of falls. Loss of traction occurs when the ground upon which the person is stepping is wet or slippery, and the person's feet fly out from under them. Loss of traction can include tripping, especially over uneven surfaces such as sidewalks, curbs, or floor elevations.

In Chapter 12, I said I had fallen outside of a movie theater as a result of an uneven crack in the handicap area. That fall resulted in the fractured patella. Surgery, recovery, and physical therapy were all necessary because of that fall.

A fall can occur because a person's reflexes (automatic stimuli in the environment) have changed. As people age, reflexes slow down. Since aging slows a person's reaction time, it makes it harder to regain their balance following sudden movements or a shift in body weight.

Changes in muscle and body fat also play a role according to the National Institute of Health. As people get older they lose muscle mass because they have become less active. Loss of muscle mass, especially in the legs, reduces a person's strength to the point where they may even need assistance getting up out of a chair. With aging is the loss of body fat that has cushioned and protected bony area, such as the hips. Loss of cushioning affects the soles of the feet, which upsets the person's ability to balance. All of this plays a major role in falling.

As I have stated several times in this book, my doctors have told me to swim every day to build up the muscle strength to protect my bones when I do fall. I was finally able to purchase an above-ground pool, and if you have a pool, start swimming now as prevention. Help your muscles and bones now. It can make a drastic difference later in life.

The NIH also claims vision changes increase the risk of falls. This can be corrected. If a person wears glasses that are bifocal or trifocal, depth perception can be altered. People wearing bifocals or trifocals must practice looking straight ahead and lowering their head. For many, vision changes cannot be completely corrected, again raising the risk of a fall.

The force of a fall (how a person lands) plays a major role on determining whether a person will fracture or not. The greater the distance of the hip bone to the floor, the greater the risk of fracturing a hip. The angle at which a person falls is also important. Falling sideways or straight down is more risky than falling backwards according to the NIH.

Reflexes and changes in posture that break a fall can reduce the risk of fracturing a bone as a result of a fall. Earlier in this book I mentioned when I fall how I try to think quickly to twist or turn in attempt to avoid another fracture. Below is a diagram of the fall triangle.

The Fracture Triangle[19]

This Fracture Triangle includes the following three factors that play a role in the breaking of a bone:

Fall

Force   **Fragility**

The **Fall** Itself

The **Force** and Direction of the Fall

The **Fragility** of the Bone(s) That Take the Impact

---

[19] This chart is courtesy of the National Institute of Health - Osteoporosis and Related Bone Disease. .

According to the National Institute of Health - Osteoporosis and Related Bone Diseases:

Did You Know?

• More than 90% of hip fractures are associated with osteoporsis?

• Nine out of ten hip fractures in older Americans are the result of a fall?

• Individuals who have a hip fracture are 5-20% more likely to die in the first year following that injury than others in this age group?

• For those living independently before a hip fracture, 15-25% will still be in long-term care institutions a year after their fracture?

• Most falls happen to women in their homes in the afternoon?

Remember it is important to consult your doctor before making any type of diagnosis or starting a treatment. Your doctor knows what is best for you and can monitor changes. Be good to yourself. If you do not take care of yourself- no one else will. You can be given guidelines, medication, and therapy exercises to do, but only you can follow through.

Healthy Diet Builds Healthy Bones

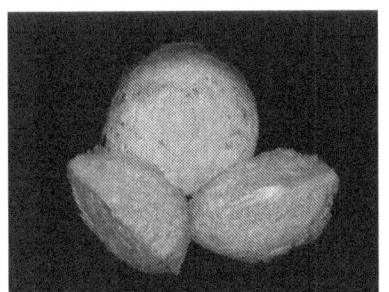 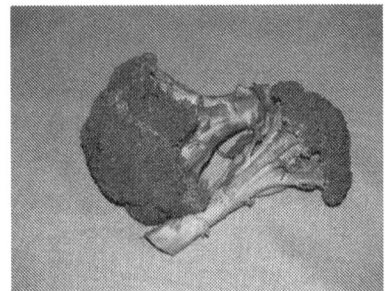

Leafy Green Vegetables

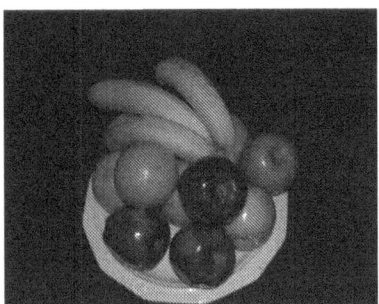

Fresh Fruits

Healthy Diet Builds Healthy Bones Continued

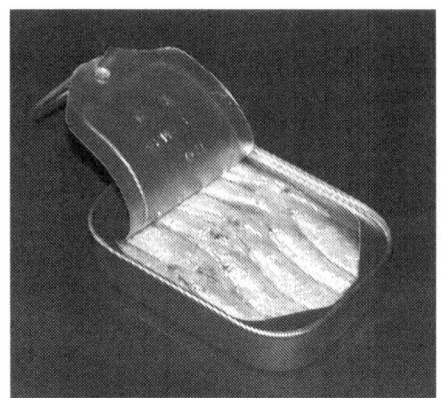

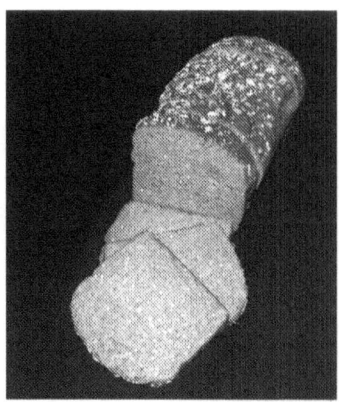

Seafood   **Calcium-enriched Bread**

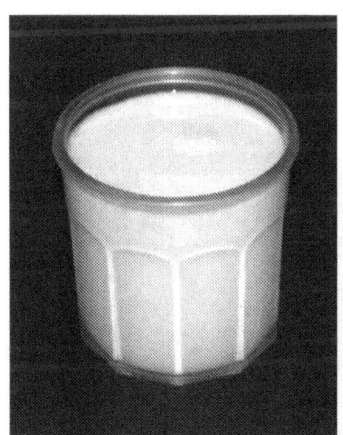

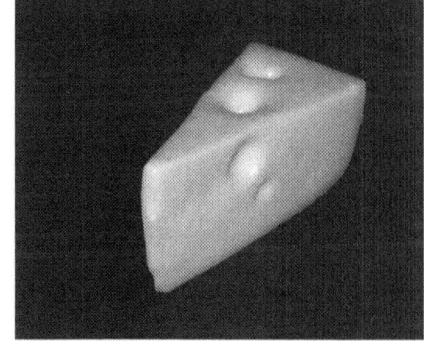

Dairy Products

Exercise Is Just As Important For Healthy Bones

Below are a few examples. Be sure to consult your doctor prior to starting a new exercise program.

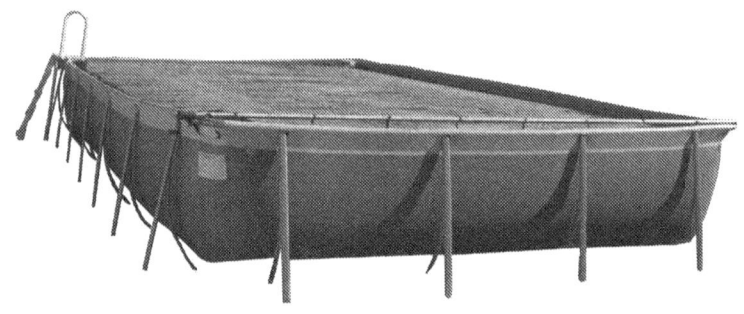

Swimming

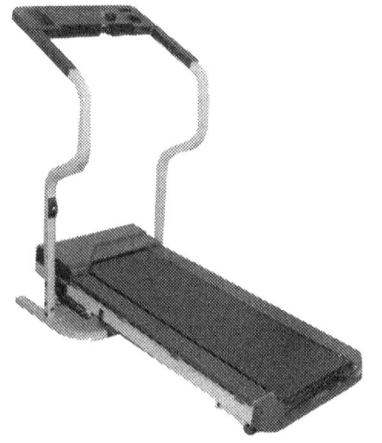

Walking or Jogging

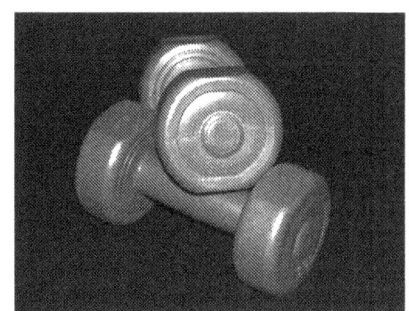

Lifting Weights

Author's Final Note

As I sat down to begin the task of writing this book, I never realized how difficult it would become. Writing the first one-third of the book was rather simple. Discussing the health issues of my childhood and early adult years was not that hard. But the second-third of the book became a very haunting time for me.

Once I was diagnosed with severe osteoporosis in 1991, I had to face the reality of the disease and how the rest of my life would be affected because of it. I had to understand that my family would also be affected and their support would be crucial in my acceptance. That was a difficult time as I tried to deal with the reality of what was happening. I did a better job at being in denial.

The most difficult and challenging times while writing the book "Living Day To Day With Severe Osteoporosis" came as I relived each major fracture, surgery when it was necessary and the physical therapy that followed. I had to dig deep within myself to recall the extent of the pain, the frustration at my limitations, the discouragement that I would never heal and be "normal" again, and knowing the hell I would go through during the recovery process and at times wishing I would not have to reach that point. Physical therapy was definitely that tough.

Each injury I wrote about was difficult. It was like I had the fracture all over again. As each healing process was signed off from the doctor over-seeing me, I would turn that page and move on until the next broken bone. Now I was bringing "back to life" not one but every major fracture and their consequences. It left me emotionally drained.

To be completely honest in my medical journey I had to face my demons and openly talk about them. That also included all the denial. In the back of mind, I always felt the doctors were telling me how bad it was, to scare me, so I would be careful and not become permanently disabled. Then in December of 2004, when the doctors gave me my latest bone density test results and said I was a liability to my employer or any employer for that matter, I realized they were not scaring me from getting that bad. I was that bad! It had happened! Paralysis was the only life-changing event I had yet to face. And I will fight it with all that is in me.

So now the only fight I have left is the big one, and that is to try and be careful and not become a paraplegic or quadriplegic. I do not want to end up in a wheelchair for the rest of my life. My doctor at the Mayo Clinic said I would have both of my hips replaced by the time I was 45. Well, I turned fifty-one in December of 2006, and I still have my own hips. That gives me strength and hope.

So please see your doctor and get a bone density test. Start prevention treatment now. Do not travel down my path. It's painful and discouraging knowing there are no bright lights at the end of the tunnel. Love yourself enough to do it. Love your family enough to do it. And if it happens — know that you can survive. I am! I am surviving as I live day to day with severe osteoporosis.

About the Author

The book "Living Day To Day With Severe Osteoporosis" is Alice V. Roberts debut in book publishing. However, Alice has written several short articles for her local newspaper as an advocate for the National Osteoporosis Foundation.

Alice was diagnosed by the Mayo Clinic in Scottsdale, Arizona with severe osteoporosis at the age of 35, and at age 49 was placed on permanent disability due to her bone density scores (-4.5: results that would have been expected from a woman in her mid-90's). She has broken most major bones more than once, had fractures that required major surgeries and physical therapy, and has approximately 20 rib fractures a year (just from sneezing, coughing, and moving the wrong way). She must use a cane and cannot lift over five pounds for the rest of her life.

As an advocate for the National Osteoporosis Foundation, Alice has formed a support group in her community that meets monthly. The National Osteoporosis Foundation provides all information and materials for the meetings, which are free of charge and open to the public. Alice has also built a web site (http://www.alicevroberts.com) that provides information regarding her book, the support group, a link to the National Osteoporosis Foundation, a Post Office for e-mails, and other informative pages for those interested in or suffering from osteoporosis.

Due to her age and severity, it is Alice's mission to make people aware of the disease osteoporosis, what its causes are, and how someone can prevent from going down the road she has traveled with osteoporosis. And now at age 51, as her book is being published, she realizes her work has just begun in the fight against this disease. If just one person can be helped Alice feels her endeavor will have been successful.

www.ingramcontent.com/pod-product-compliance
Lightning Source LLC
Chambersburg PA
CBHW061305280526
45784CB00002B/906